"This is an amazing book, a veritable treasure trove of information for cancer patients, for their friends and families.

It is a very detailed description of the various cancers that can afflict us all and the various approaches to their treatment.

It is written by a lay person who, after a struggle for many years with complex biological therapy and chemotherapy, has conquered a form of chronic leukaemia.

He has devoted a decade of his life to finding out more about cancer and how such knowledge can help individual patients cope with the fear and difficulties of their treatments.

In this book he offers a gift of knowledge and understanding that makes the struggle easier and perhaps more worthwhile for patients."

PROFESSOR RICHARD FOX, FRACP, PhD, DIRECTOR OF THE DEPARTMENT OF CLINICAL HEMATOLOGY AND MEDICAL ONCOLOGY, ROYAL MELBOURNE HOSPITAL, PRESIDENT, AUSTRALIAN CANCER SOCIETY 1995-98

"Joel Nathan has created an invaluable survival guide which allows people affected by cancer an opportunity to regain a sense of control over their lives."

ROBIN POPE, ONCOLOGY EDUCATION CONSULTANT, FREEMASONS HOSPITAL, MELBOURNE

"At last, a book that is readable, relevant, and comprehensive enough to appeal to all of those who have cancer, have had cancer or who care for those with cancer. I cannot recommend this too highly."

PROFESSOR MICHAEL A. QUINN, DIRECTOR OF THE ONCOLOGY/DYSPLASIA UNIT, ROYAL WOMEN'S HOSPITAL, MELBOURNE

"Joel's knowledge parallels his life experience – he is now sharing it with others. This is an excellent consultant guide for the patient."

DR JOHN SULLIVAN, HEMATOLOGIST/ONCOLOGIST

To

the Good Doctor

John Sullivan

What to do when they say "It's cancer."

Joel Nathan

ALLEN & UNWIN

Purchase of this book in Australia contributes funds to the Australian Cancer Society

First published in 1998 by
Allen & Unwin
9 Atchison Street
St Leonards NSW 1590
Australia

Phone: (61 2) 8425 0100
Fax: (61 2) 9906 2218
E-mail: frontdesk@allen-unwin.com.au
Web: http://www.allen-unwin.com.au

National Library of Australia
Cataloguing-in-Publication entry:

Nathan, Joel, 1940–.
What to do when they say "It's cancer" : a survivor's guide.
ISBN 1 86448 635 X
1. Cancer – Treatment. I. Title.

616.994

Set in 11.7pt Granjon by J&M Typesetting
Cover and text design by Ruth Grüner
Cover image by Thayer Syme, courtesy of Austral International
Author photograph on back cover by René Nathan
Index by Russell Brooks
Printed by Australian Print Group, Maryborough, Victoria

3 5 7 9 10 8 6 4 2

9/2000

Caroline,
"Hope is a good thing,
maybe the best of things
and good things never die!"

acknowledgements *with love,*

ß

Many people contributed to the writing of this book, directly and indirectly, and I am grateful to them for their assistance. Foremost were those cancer patients and their families who shared their deepest thoughts with me in times of great distress as well as joy.

I was supported by my family and friends who tiptoed around me as I worked on the book. In particular, I would like to thank my wife, René, for her unfailing love, support and wise counsel in what turned out be a much longer-than-expected writing schedule.

The first person I showed this manuscript to was Professor Richard Fox, Director of the Department of Clinical Hematology and Medical Oncology at the Royal Melbourne Hospital, who affirmed that a book like this was long overdue and much needed by patients, health professionals and medical students alike. I have had wonderful support and shared the journey with some other very special people, including Dr John Sullivan, whom I thank for his advice and patience in checking and re-checking key medical aspects; Professor Paul Bunn, Jnr, Director of the University of Colorado Cancer Center, President of the International Association for the Study of Lung Cancer, recent Chairman of the FDA Oncology Drugs Advisory Committee, for his guidance and ideas, particularly those dealing with doctor-patient issues and with alternative treatments; Professor Michael Quinn, Director of the Oncology/Dysplasia Unit at the Royal Women's Hospital, Melbourne, for providing pithy comments and helpful tips throughout the book; Robin Pope, Oncology Education Consultant at the Freemasons Hospital, Melbourne, for her practical suggestions, ongoing encouragement and friendship; Dr Yvonne Greenberg for her recommendations and sage counsel; Pat Dobson, indefatigable co-ordinator of Social Services, Anti-Cancer Council of Victoria, for her friendship, counsel and understanding; Cynthia Holland, Senior Oncology Clinician (Social Work), Royal Women's Hospital, Melbourne, for her encouragement and passionate discussions, particularly regarding the delicate issue of children; Jill Storey, Clinical Nurse Consultant, Royal Women's Hospital, Melbourne, for her down-to-earth advice on coping with side effects of treatment; Professor Robert Burton, Director of the Anti-Cancer Council of Victoria, for his generous support and suggestions for this book; Graham Giles and Doreen Akkerman of the Anti-Cancer Council of Victoria, for help with statistics and resources; Patrick Condron of the Brownless Medical Library, Melbourne University, for helping me to double-check the medical references.

Not least, I wish to thank my agent, Jill Hickson, who first saw what I hoped to achieve with this book, for her faith in it, her encouragement and advice; to Sophie Lance of Hickson and Associates for her practical guidance; and my publishing team at Allen and Unwin – Jackie Yowell whose enthusiasm for the book was matched only by her determination to make it amenable to as many readers as possible; Sarah Brenan, my editor, whose advice and worn-down pencils helped make the book light enough to be held by even the weakest of patients; Jenn Lane and Ruth Grüner, who helped make the book so attractive.

Of course, there would have been no book without the life-saving efforts of Dr John Sullivan, Professor Richard Fox, Dr Emmanuel Manolas, Dr Saibal Kar, and the life-preserving surgical skills of Mr John Goldblatt and Mr Lawrence Simpson.

My model of the good doctor throughout this book was Dr John Sullivan, whose compassion, sense of humour, superb diagnostic skills and determination to leave no stone unturned are attested by thousands of grateful patients.

Finally, I want to thank my sons Gregory, Trevor and Brian for their unswerving love through two cancer crises.

Thank you.
In light and peace,

Joel Nathan

foreword

Cancer will develop in one in three Americans during their life-time. No other single event is likely to have a greater impact on their lives. Yet no one is prepared for the dramatic and devastating effects of cancer on their own life or on the life of loved ones.

What to do when they say 'It's cancer' is an outstanding primer for those who develop cancer, as well as for their loved ones. It is written by a true expert; namely, an individual who has not only experienced cancer himself, but has also worked with cancer health professionals, cancer patients and their families. The author, Joel Nathan, describes his own struggle with complex therapies, decisions, highs and lows and uncertainties of outcome. He provides practical advice on the selection of physicians and therapies, understanding feelings, communication, caring and living in the face of death. I recommend this book for anyone diagnosed with cancer, their family members and friends. It should help them adjust, face their problems and make the right choices.

PROFESSOR PAUL A. BUNN, JNR, M.D.,
DIRECTOR OF THE UNIVERSITY OF
COLORADO CANCER CENTER, PRESIDENT OF
THE INTERNATIONAL ASSOCIATION FOR THE
STUDY OF LUNG CANCER, PAST-PRESIDENT OF
THE ASSOCIATION OF AMERICAN CANCER
INSTITUTES, BOARD OF DIRECTORS TO
AMERICAN SOCIETY OF CLINICAL ONCOLOGY,
RECENT CHAIRMAN OF FDA'S ONCOLOGY DRUGS
ADVISORY COMMITTEE

contents

Part One

diagnosis

'cancer'

one

if we only knew...

'While there's hope, there's life.'

JOEL NATHAN

When I was a child I used to have a recurrent nightmare. I was being chased by a lion. No matter how hard I tried to run, my legs wouldn't move. I felt trapped.

Nothing recaptured that caught feeling more vividly than my doctor saying, 'It's cancer', 43 years later.

At once all the desperate terror of my childhood nightmare returned: *'This feels like a bad dream. It can't be happening to me. I'll wake up soon and it'll be over.'* But I knew this was not a dream. I could feel the blood drain from my face, my stomach contract; everything went quiet.

When I unfroze, I thrashed around, looking for a way out of this nightmare. At the time, there was no treatment to cure my rare form of leukemia. I searched everywhere for a way out, but every direction I took led me back to the same bad dream. The full story of my battle to survive the prognosis that I had less than three months to live is told in my first book, *Time of my Life*.

When I had recovered, I decided to write the kind of book I wished had been available to me when I was first diagnosed with cancer – a guide that would tell me all the things I had to find out the hard way, the things doctors never mentioned, the things it was nobody's responsibility to tell me about.

- How do you go about getting a second opinion?
- How do you break the bad news to your family and friends – and especially your children?
- How do you choose the right doctor for you?

- How do you find the best treatment for your particular type of cancer, and for your particular needs?
- How do you build confidence to make your own choices?
- How can you and your family best handle the practical and psychological stresses of your changed life?
- How do you maintain optimism and hold despair at bay?
- How do you find a meaning to life while facing your own death?
- How can you conquer your fear of dying?

I wanted to offer others a book that would take the fear out of cancer, and maximise the chances of survival by providing practical advice for meeting the medical and emotional demands of cancer in the best way possible. In doing so, I have drawn not only on my own experience but that of countless others.

I completed the draft of this book five days after undergoing surgery for lung cancer. I am determined to survive cancer again.

In the twelve years between my two different cancers, I have counselled people with various life-threatening illnesses. I have addressed support groups and gatherings of doctors and nurses. I have researched every aspect of cancer – its causes, cures, physical and social effects, emotional and spiritual impact. Using my own databases, the Internet and the advice of consulting doctors, I started a company to help people find out more about their illnesses and treatments. As I complete this book, and apart from counselling cancer patients, I am working with a health-promoting palliative care unit and a cancer association to develop and promote cancer support, health and death education, and survival skills.

This book grew out of my experiences in survival. It is essentially about how your own resourcefulness and spirit can enhance your survival – *for however long*. When you are despairing, it is often the stories of others suffering the same experience that can inspire, guide and comfort you. But first let me retell my story, as it reveals the context for much I have learned about surviving cancer.

It began in the summer of 1982 with a pain in my right shoulder. At first I ascribed it to my strenuous exercise schedule. I managed to ignore the pain for a few weeks, but when it became unbearable, I went to see my general practitioner. He thought I had strained a muscle, so he sent me to a physiotherapist. After weeks of deep massage, manipulation, ultrasound and cortisone injections, he referred me to an orthopedic surgeon. He, in turn, could make no clear diagnosis.

I was now convinced that my increasing tiredness was simply due to the relentless pain, so I visited an acupuncturist. After several weeks, with my distress still unrelieved, my GP's partner was less concerned about my painful shoulder than my paleness. Mumbling 'possibly anemia' under his breath, he sent me to a hematologist, a specialist in blood disorders. In an attempt to find out why I was now having night sweats and why my blood counts kept falling, he sent me for a blood test once a week for the next eight months. Meanwhile, I tried to bury myself in work.

I didn't realise it at the time, but working longer hours provided me with an explanation for my growing tiredness, while my giving up all sports gave me an excuse for my expanding midriff. Out of fear of what they might say, I didn't challenge my doctors' opinion, nor did I consider asking for a second one.

Eventually, the specialist suggested I have a bone marrow biopsy. The result was inconclusive. In the end, I endured no less than sixteen of these agonising procedures.

CAT (Computer Aided Tomography) scans and more blood tests followed. Still no one could diagnose my problem. The night sweats had become worse. I changed my pyjamas and the bedclothes several times a night. When these ran out, I slept on towels.

The months dragged on. Small lumps started to develop in my groin and my armpits. When I came out in boils, I was tested for fevers found in countries I had never visited.

In late 1983 I underwent a second bone-marrow biopsy. Two days later, my doctor called me in and said, 'At last! We have a name for it. It's an extremely rare form of cancer called hairy cell leukemia.'

'Is it benign?' I asked.

'No,' he said. 'It's malignant.'

The pit of doom engulfed me.

'How long do I have?' I asked, outwardly composed.

'I can't say,' he said. 'But if we remove your spleen, we could buy you a little time.'

My second question was, 'Will the operation save my life?'

'There is no cure,' he replied. 'But I have made arrangements with a top surgeon to remove your spleen. You should be home before Christmas.'

The moment he told me he had made arrangements for surgery without consulting me, all my survival instincts were aroused. I decided to get a second opinion.

I couldn't get an appointment with an oncologist, a cancer specialist, for two weeks. My acupuncturist opened the door to an endless line of people offering a range of alternative treatments. By the time I went for a second opinion from the oncologist, I'd discovered meditation, changed my diet, attended church and lined up appointments with several healers.

The oncologist confirmed the initial diagnosis. As for the pain in my shoulder, he was surprised that no one had told me it was a referred pain from my spleen. Two days later, I called my doctor and told him to cancel the operation. He was not impressed, and told me so.

'I went to a lot of trouble to set it up,' he said.

By now, my night sweats had become more severe, my tiredness a constant drain. I began to experience severe headaches. The lumps in my groin were swollen and most uncomfortable. My spleen was growing larger and more painful day by day.

I became convinced that alternative medicine offered more hope. For more than a year I followed the regimens of some well-known alternative therapists – Gerson, Isserls, Kelly, Breuss and Wigmore – and some obscure ones. I was treated by spiritual healers, numerologists, a hypnotherapist, a clairvoyant, a world-famous psychic surgeon from the Philippines and a homeopath from India. I tried Chinese medicine – including acupuncture, poultices, herbs and heated suction cups on my back. I tried homeopathy, macrobiotics, naturopathy and visualisation. I consumed vast amounts of vitamins, especially vitamin C; at one stage, I was taking 40 g a day. I bought a non-centrifugal juice extractor and drank thirteen juices a day made from vegetables, wheat grass, raw liver and carrots.

The paraphernalia of alternative medicine had me mesmerised. Nothing was too far-fetched to try. I twirled crystals over my food to determine if they were right for me, and placed a broom under my bed to align me with the earth's magnetic forces. I ate organically grown vegetables, avoided cooking in aluminium pots. I tested for food allergies. I tried various fasts, exotic herbs, took colonic irrigations and coffee enemas.

I believed that my optimism could keep me afloat, that my determination would steer me through these troubled waters. I meditated for several hours daily, joined a cancer support group, and read extensively. Staying alive was exhausting – and very expensive. I had stopped working to devote myself fully to my recovery. It was not an easy decision; in the end, it broke my marriage.

Despite all my efforts and my conviction that I was on the right course, the evidence pointed the other way. My blood counts continued to fall. The night sweats continued, and my spleen grew larger. I was able to walk only two or three paces before stopping to catch my breath and allow my heart to stop pounding. My gums – and later, my nose – began to bleed spontaneously; I would wake to find my pillow soaked in blood. My headaches became more severe. My expanding spleen hurt more and more, jamming up against my stomach so I could not eat a full meal. Eventually, I subsisted by sipping juices and snacking. I had also turned bright yellow from carrot juice.

This presented many unforeseen problems. I had reluctantly agreed with my wife's decision not to tell our children about my illness. In order to ensure there would be no breach in this wall of denial, we kept the news from friends and workmates alike for almost a year. Everyone thought I had jaundice and could not understand why I was taking so long to recover. The most serious consequence of this decision was the effect on my sons. It has taken me a long time to heal the wounds of lost trust. I learnt how unwise it is to protect your loved ones from reality.

A year after my diagnosis, I suffered a retinal hemorrhage. Later that day, I received my first platelet transfusion. Despite determined optimism, my life now became dependent on full blood transfusions every week, and platelet transfusions whenever my gum and nose bleeds could not be stanched. At the same time, stories about a new and deadly virus, AIDS, began to appear in the newspapers. Contaminated blood was implicated in many of the new cases. Each transfusion became a game of Russian roulette.

Each bone marrow biopsy revealed an increase in the number of hairy cells. Platelet transfusions were becoming less effective. The consensus of medical opinion was that I was likely to die within three months – most probably from a brain hemorrhage or severe infection.

A near-death experience, complete with a tunnel of light and clouds of love, helped me cope with my fear of death. I was now living by the day, finding peace in meditation, solace in the ageless insights of spiritual teachings.

But the reality of my situation was that my spleen was now 28 cm long – a normal spleen cannot be felt. My hemoglobin count was 4.5 – normal is 13.5-18.0. My white cell count was 0.6 – normal is 4.0-11.0. My platelet count was 9 000 – normal is 150 000-400 000. I was running on water. I could do nothing now except pray for a miracle.

It appeared a week later in *Time* magazine. In the 1 July 1985 issue, I came across an article about a new drug – interferon – being trialled in the USA. Interferon is a naturally occurring substance and forms an essential component of the body's own immune system. I felt goosebumps on my arms as I read that the disease for which interferon had achieved remarkable success was a rare and uniformly fatal form of cancer: hairy cell leukemia.

I called my specialist and told him of my find. Thanks to his efforts, two weeks later I became the first person in Australia to receive this wonder drug. Today, interferon is a front-line drug against hairy cell leukemia as well as a number of other once-fatal cancers. Nonetheless, the treatment proved almost as uncomfortable as the symptoms of the disease itself.

Tests to ensure the safety of trial drugs are extensive. Interferon was no exception. I had to undergo more bone-marrow biopsies, bone scans, blood tests, cardiographs, liver ultrasound scans, chest X-rays and body CAT scans. I was injected with radioactive dyes and scrutinised on monitor screens in subterranean rooms. I was X-rayed after swallowing porridges of barium and mixtures of alkalis and acids to make me fizz. I was X-rayed standing up, lying down and upside down.

At that time, no one knew what the most effective dose should be. My initial dose was four times what was later considered optimal. For the first few weeks my temperature hovered around 40° C. I had all the symptoms of unrelenting influenza: my teeth chattered, my head hurt. Two large fans helped to cool me down, two hot water bottles and several blankets were used to keep me warm. My blood counts fell even lower, so I had to receive innumerable blood and platelet transfusions to keep me going. To say I felt wretched is an understatement.

When I left hospital after almost three weeks, no one knew whether the treatment had worked or not. It didn't matter to me: I felt as if I had been granted a life pardon.

I gave myself injections for the next three years, during which time my symptoms slowly receded. It was a time to heal, a time to reflect on what I had been through, a time to decide what I wanted to do with the rest of my life – however long that might be.

I began to prepare notes for my first book, worked as a volunteer with cancer patients and then, after further study, began counselling. It was a time of hope, exploration and a new appreciation of life. To cap it all, my eldest son graduated as a doctor.

It was also a time of learning. I realised that not only was there much about cancer I still didn't know, but that most other people knew even less. It seemed that doctors were either reluctant or unable to communicate with their patients, and that people, by and large, are given little guidance on what to do when they are diagnosed with cancer.

These experiences began to crowd my thoughts, and so I began writing my first book, *Time of My Life*, sharing what I had learned and beginning to explore the themes that have crystallised in this one. (Readers who are interested can obtain copies of it from me via the publisher of this book.)

Partly out of my desire to learn as much as I could about cancer, and partly because I was still hopeful of finding some new treatment to cure me completely, I continued reading the most up-to-date medical journals and textbooks.

About a year later, I read an article in the authoritative *New England Journal of Medicine* about a new drug being trialled in California. The drug was 2-chloro-deoxy-adenosine, or 2-CDA. According to the initial results, doctors had achieved remarkable success in treating people with hairy cell leukemia and non-Hodgkin's lymphoma.

I contacted the institute which had developed the drug and obtained more information about it. Successful as interferon had been, it was clear that this drug broke new ground. I was determined to take part in the trial even though, as I soon found out, I was ineligible because my blood counts were too high for the baseline required by the trial. To become eligible, I would have had to turn the clock back five years.

Undeterred, I approached a well-known professor of oncology in Australia and gave him all the information I had gathered. I then asked him to help to import the drug from the USA for me. Although interferon had saved my life, my blood counts were still not ideal. In 2-CDA I saw a chance of complete recovery.

'I'll do what I can,' he said. 'But government red tape is bound to get in the way.'

I did not feel confident when I left his office.

Two days later, at one o'clock in the morning, he called to say that the National Cancer Institute in Washington had agreed to include me in its trial and was sending 2-CDA by express mail. I don't know who was more excited – the professor or me.

Ten days later we started the treatment. For seven days I received a continuous infusion of the new drug. There were no side effects, except from the champagne we drank to celebrate. I was confident about the outcome. Within a few months, my blood counts had stabilised. It seemed we had won not only one more battle, but the war.

With a sense of having gained a more secure lease on life, I devoted all my working time to writing and counselling. I married a second time. I watched my other two sons graduate, the middle in science and commerce, the youngest also as a doctor. It was a wonderful time of easy optimism.

Then, in the summer of 1995-96, my childhood nightmare returned. For a few weeks I had been swimming in an attempt to regain my fitness. No matter how hard I tried, I could not increase the number of laps I was swimming. I felt as if I were paddling in slow motion through a vat of treacle. I persisted for a while, but there was no improvement. I contacted my cardiologist who suggested I undergo an angiogram to check my heart. A week later, as I lay waiting for this procedure, Fate intervened. I was advised that my physician had injured his back and that I should make another appointment for a time when he had recovered. My physician's assistant asked me when I had last had an X-ray of my chest.

'Why?' I asked. I knew that a chest X-ray was not part of an angiogram routine.

'Your liver is slightly enlarged. I think we should check you out.'

The following day I was X-rayed and diagnosed with non-small-cell lung cancer – a type that rarely responds to either chemotherapy or radiotherapy and for which early diagnosis and surgery were the only hope of long-term survival.

In my first encounter with cancer, the symptoms of the disease had been worse than the treatment; this time it was the other way around. Tiredness apart, I had experienced no other symptoms prior to surgery; but after an operation to remove the middle lobe of my right lung, I found myself in the most unbearable pain. The surgeons had to cut not only the nerves and lining of my lung, but also one rib under my shoulder blade. While they were retracting my rib cage, another rib broke. Every time I breathed, I felt as if someone were scraping the inside of my lung with broken glass. I meditated, visualised, and prayed for relief from my pain. Morphine would have provided blessed relief, but due to my heart condition, it would also have killed me. I gritted my teeth. Thirteen days after the operation, I left the hospital. I had a book to finish.

So what have I learned from two encounters with cancer?

Both experiences have taught me that while you can't always change the situations in which you find yourself, you can change your response to them; you can see them as a profound experience in living rather than a nightmare over which you have no control. My cancers compelled me to rearrange my priorities, learn new coping skills, re-examine my relationships with people – and with God. Surviving cancer has been the most spiritually rewarding time of my life. My prospects of recovery improved from the moment I realised that my physical state was inextricably linked to my psychological and spiritual recovery. The chances of survival were multiplied from the moment I took an active role in bringing these elements together. Both experiences also taught me the value of true friends.

Most people don't know much about cancer until they have to, when they are faced with the diagnosis for themselves or for a loved one. Faced with conflicting advice and the pressures of relating to all those affected by your illness, you need a guide to help you up the mountain (for cancer is a mountain) and down the other side. I hope that this book can be that guide.

two

understanding and confirming your diagnosis

‿

'There is always more than one answer –
[the answer] depends on the question.'

VIKTOR FRANKL

Even if you have been ill for some time and half expect the worst, it is difficult to shield yourself from the impact of your doctor saying, 'You've got cancer.' Whatever the exact diagnosis, whatever your age and confidence, you are likely to have a shock reaction – 'diagnosis shock', you might call it – and you will need all your inner resources to hold yourself together. The best thing you can do for yourself at this stage is to call a halt, make space and time to adjust.

Take time to absorb and consider

There is a limit to what you can absorb in the deafening silence following the doctor's pronouncement, and what you did take in may have been softened by a doctor trying to break the news gently. Give yourself time to double-check the diagnosis and your under-standing of it, time to clarify the short- and long-term prognosis, time to realise the implications for you and your family. To stop your-self being overwhelmed by the rush of events, pause for at least a day. Your cancer took a long time to get to the point where it com-mands your undivided attention, so you don't have to make any snap decisions about it now. Rarely does anyone die overnight from cancer.

If your doctor hasn't made an appointment for you to return, ask for one, so you can double-check on what he said and ask follow-up questions. (I've listed some useful questions later on.) No one should expect you to make a life-saving decision and consider all your options at a single sitting. You need time to regain your composure, gather your thoughts, and consider your options. You need to gather as much information as you can – and you can't do so effectively if you are rushed. Your doctor should support you in this, even if takes repeated consultations with him.

Take time to consider your doctor's advice on treatment. One doctor may be conservative about trying out a new treatment, another may be over-zealous. If your doctor wants to conquer your cancer at all costs, he may subject you to every treatment he knows – without regard to its impact on your quality of life. He may believe that there is no way to cure your disease, yet still put you under the knife or give you an intense course of chemotherapy or radiotherapy. Being treated to death may not be what you have in mind.

Your doctor puts unnecessary pressure on you when, by virtue of diagnosing your disease, he assumes he has the automatic right to decide what treatment is best, and whether this should start immediately.

If you rush to start treatment immediately, you may discover later that a different procedure would have been more effective, or that your disease was not as critical as you thought; or that the treatment you thought would cure you of your disease was only able to alleviate your symptoms.

Take your time to absorb and consider what you were told. To stay in control, you have to be active – not reactive. You need to act not on impulse, but according to a deliberate and well-planned course of action.

It may take several days to come to grips with what has happened and make rational choices about how to contend with it.

Make sure you understand

It is most unlikely that you will remember or correctly interpret everything your doctor told you. For example, you may have interpreted your doctor's words to mean that there is no urgency to start treatment when in fact there is. Your understanding may be that there is no treatment when it is in fact readily available.

Your ability to take in what he has said may be affected for a number of reasons:

- If you have undergone extensive tests, you may be tired. Added to your anxiety and your fears, this would reduce your alertness and your ability to concentrate.

- You were too shocked to take in what your doctor said. No matter how well-prepared you were, if your doctor used words like 'cancer', 'malignant', or 'terminal', the buzz of fear in your ears may have prevented you from hearing anything else.

  Many people who have had a heart attack or cancer claim that their doctors never informed them about their diagnosis, the suggested treatment plan, or what the likely outcome might be, even when there is ample evidence that they were clearly told.[1]

- Your doctor may not be a good communicator. He may have confused you by using words such as 'splenomegaly', 'cannula', 'thoracotomy' or 'clonal myelo-proliferation'. Some doctors resort to med-speak, not necessarily to impress, but in order to make themselves feel more comfortable.

  Others will present you with a load of facts and feel they have done their duty, not realising that being overwhelmed with *too much* information may raise your anxiety levels even higher.

- If your doctor told you the news while you were in hospital, there's every chance that his hurried schedule prevented him taking all the time needed to make sure you understood all the implications.

- Your doctor may have been on an emotional 'low' that day for reasons of his own; treating cancer can be very demanding. If you had been his patient for some time, he might have felt so distressed he stumbled over his words, or talked about other things in the hope you would read between the lines.

- Your unexpressed fears may influence what you believe you were told. In a fearful state you may only hear what you expected to hear.

A good doctor will make sure you understand the diagnosis. You cannot be expected to make an informed choice if he doesn't. But unless you actually say you don't comprehend what you're being told – and unless your doctor keeps checking to make sure you do – you may only get half the story. Speak up. With so much at stake, you can't afford to be reticent.

The dangers of misunderstanding

Misunderstanding starts when a doctor says 'treatment', and you hear 'cure'; when he says 'inoperable' and you hear 'untreatable'. When he says you have a 'treatable disease', he may mean he can picture you back at work in six weeks; you may hear the same words and believe it is only just treatable.

Your doctor needs to be extremely precise with the words, gestures and body language he uses. At the same time, you need to be sure you don't misinterpret any of his actions. This was illustrated by Liz, a cancer patient who came to me for counselling.

Liz went to her radiologist complaining of pain in her right thigh. He had earlier treated her for lung cancer and was concerned that her disease might have spread. He sent her for X-rays. Upon finding a small growth on the bone, he treated her with a further short course of radiotherapy. A few weeks afterwards, she returned to him for a follow-up examination. Whichever part of her leg he touched, she winced with pain.

Afterwards she called me, extremely distressed.

'He doesn't seem sure whether it's worth continuing with treatment or not,' she said. 'I think he feels it's hopeless.'

I suggested she call him to double-check what he had said. Her relief was unbounded when he told her she had certainly mis-heard him. Liz thought he had said, 'Well, will we keep on with the treatment?', but in fact he had said, 'Well, we'll have to keep on with the treatment,' feeling sure that further treatment was vital to ensure success – as it was. A few months later a scan, and the absence of any symptoms, revealed that her cancer was in remission.

The importance of asking questions

Many people find it difficult to question the authority of doctors. Be careful if you find yourself saying things like:

'I suppose I'll have to do what my doctor says.'

'You can't mess around with cancer.'

'I'm sure my doctor knows what he's talking about.'

'I'd be too embarrassed to ask again. I mean, he did tell me.'

Try not to be swayed by such feelings. If you are, you are unlikely to make an informed decision.

'But,' you may say, 'I don't know what questions to ask.'

Any question you have concerning your life is valid.

As a guide, I've listed all the questions I and others have found it useful to ask. Write them down or take this book with you. It would be a pity to remember all the things you wanted to ask *after* you have left your doctor's rooms.

If you feel awkward about reading out a whole list of questions, take someone you trust with you to give you moral support – or to ask these questions on your behalf. Take your spouse, your companion, a parent, an adult child, a close friend, to accompany you on your next visit. Apart from their support, they can be a further check afterwards of what your doctor said.

Questions to ask your doctor

- Are you absolutely sure I have cancer?
- Have you performed all the tests necessary to confirm your diagnosis?
- What type of cancer do I have?
- What parts of my body has it affected?
- What more can you tell me about my disease?
- What type of treatment do you believe is best for my disease?
- What would happen if I had no treatment?
- Have you treated many people with my type and stage of cancer? How successful was the outcome?
- Are you offering me the latest treatment? Are there any clinical trials under way for my particular disease?
- How long will the whole treatment program last? A week, two weeks, a month?
- How often will I receive treatment? Every day, every other day, once a week?
- If I can't cope with this (e.g., injections), is there an alternative form?
- What actually happens to me in the process of this treatment?

- What side effects am I likely to experience – and how well can you manage them? How have other people responded to it? (Don't assume too much from others' experience – everyone is different in age, fitness, lifestyle and attitude.)
- Can I have the treatment at home?
- When will I be able to return to work or carry on my hobbies?
- How costly is the treatment? Will I have to pay for it myself, and if so, how much?
- Can you continue to provide me with information about my disease and treatments, or can you direct me to where I can research them?

If your doctor has not already told you, ask him how other patients have responded to the same treatment for the same type of cancer you have. But be careful not to assume too much from this. The same treatment program may succeed with one person and fail with another – and vice versa.

If your doctor says he has seen few successful outcomes from treatment for your type of cancer, don't be afraid to say, 'Can you please refer me to someone who has treated my type of cancer before, successfully?'

In the absence of satisfactory answers to your questions, you owe it to yourself and your family to get someone else to take a fresh look at you and your case history.

Take a tape recorder

To make absolutely sure no one misinterprets what your doctor says, and to make sure all of you have all the facts, take a tape recorder with you. If you feel you're taking up your doctor's valuable time by asking him what may seem like trivial questions, you would do well to remember who is ill and who is not.

The difference between your saying, 'My doctor told me...' and saying, 'I *think* my doctor told me...' may cause you to postpone treatment when it is most inadvisable to do so. A tape recording of your discussion will remove all doubts.

Mirroring

If you're not completely sure you understand what your doctor told you, use the technique of 'mirroring' – telling your doctor what you heard him say. Mirroring does *not* mean repeating, like a parrot, what you have been told. It means restating what you have been told in your own words. For example:

DOCTOR: Three days of chemotherapy should shrink the tumor. I feel that after that, it should cause you no more problems.

MIRROR: You mean that it may shrink the tumor but you can't guarantee it?

DOCTOR: Yes.

You need to mirror everything. For example:

YOU: What do you mean by 'three days'?

DOCTOR: I mean you should have one treatment lasting about an hour each days for three consecutive days.

YOU (mirroring): So I only need to come in for an hour every day for three days, and I can go home after each treatment?

DOCTOR: Correct.

If you think your doctor will regard this approach as a waste of time, remind yourself that it is far safer to be sure than to pretend you understand. If you aren't certain of the facts, you might fill the gaps in your knowledge with speculation, leading to anxiety and confusion.

There would be fewer breakdowns in communications between doctors and patients if this simple technique were used.

Compelling yourself to use this technique has several other major benefits:

☞   You and your doctor can reflect each other's expectations.

☞   You can consider what you're doing and weigh up your options.

☞   You feel you have a more active role in saving your life.

Mirroring helps to overcome the problems that can arise through mis-reading body language. For example, you nod your head to acknowledge what you have been told, but your doctor thinks you've nodded your head in agreement with his proposed treatment plan. You fold your arms because you're trembling with fear, but your doctor assumes you've adopted a negative posture and don't wish to co-operate.

Establishing the full truth

If your doctor tells you he wants you to undergo further tests, ask him why. If your doctor is afraid to tell you that the treatment for your condition has little chance of success, sending you for more tests may only serve to help him postpone telling you the truth.

Your doctor may be fascinated by your condition and want to learn more about it. Sending you for more tests will certainly satisfy his curiosity – but it may do little to affect the course or the outcome of your treatment.

Your doctor expects you to follow his advice so he can provide you with the best help he knows. You expect your doctor to tell you whatever you need to know so you can co-operate with confidence. You may be feeling nervous because you've been waiting to hear about the results of a recent test; your doctor may be feeling uncomfortable about what he has to tell you. Neither of you will be able to meet each other's expectations, or be at ease with each other, if you fail to recognise them.

If you don't want to hear the truth, that is your choice and your right. However, if you want to retain your autonomy and take an active part in your treatment program, it is essential that you get the facts. In Australia, for example, your doctor has to tell you – even if your family asks him not to.[2]

If you have the slightest doubt about what you have been told, tackle the issue head-on, and ask your doctor, 'Have you told me everything? Have you told me the truth?'

Refusing to talk about your disease won't make it go away. If your doctor holds back from telling you the truth at the time of your diagnosis because he feels he will upset you, you're bound to feel more aggrieved when you learn about it later. In any event, refusing to tell you the truth denies you the chance to explore new possibilities – for your disease as well as yourself.

This view is echoed by Dr Elisabeth Kübler-Ross, who maintains that people cope better when they are told early on that they have a life-threatening disease. She also found that when people realise they aren't going to die overnight, the hope of living longer actually helps them live longer.

In a survey she conducted among her patients, Kübler-Ross found that the majority of people wanted their doctors to be honest with them so they could come to terms with the seriousness of their condition, and ask for more information when they felt ready to ask for it.[3]

Getting a second opinion

Many people persist with a doctor in whom they have little confidence. Among the reasons they offer is that they do not want to offend their doctor or make him feel that his professional ability is being questioned.[4] Other people are concerned about costs. There is no doubt that the more money you have, the more choice you have over medical attention and treatment. Yet if you are in the public health system and you have been diagnosed in a hospital, you can still get a second opinion. Simply ask your doctor to refer you to another doctor in the same clinic. If he refuses or suggests the clinic is too busy to accede to your request, ask the hospital administrator to act on your behalf.

If the thought of upsetting your doctor crosses your mind, perhaps you need to ask yourself what is more important: hurting his feelings or improving your chances of survival? The doctor who feels you are challenging his knowledge and experience may make these, or similar comments to you:

- 'I suppose you're free to do what you want.'
- 'If you insist, but it means I will have to send all your files to him, and we are very busy.'
- 'Leave it with me and I'll talk it over with one of my colleagues.'
- 'I can't stop you getting you getting another opinion, but I think you're wasting your time.'
- 'Don't you think I know what I'm doing?'

Don't be put off by statements like these. Your doctor may believe he is acting in your best interests, but if he tries to deter you from seeking another opinion, he is not.

The danger of this attitude is reflected in the joke:

PATIENT: Doctor, I'd like to get another opinion.

DOCTOR: OK. Let me take another guess.

To be really sure you are getting the best advice, ask your doctor to refer you to someone he has not briefed. **You need an independent second opinion – not a second first opinion.**

If you can't get the information you need through your GP, check the Resource Guide at the back of this book, or your local goods and services directory for the cancer association nearest you, then seek some advice from a counsellor.

Why you need a second opinion

The aim of getting a second opinion is *not* to prove your doctor wrong, or yourself right. If your doctor is a GP, you need to see a cancer specialist (oncologist) to confirm that the diagnosis was correct, and to explore the possibility of other, even better treatment options. Even if you have seen an oncologist, you need a second opinion to make sure you get the option best suited to you.

Few doctors outline all the options available and explain the pros and cons of each. Instead, they choose what *they* think is the most suitable option for you. In a take-it-or-leave-it atmosphere, you can feel a loss of control. Seeking a second opinion not only gives you back the reins, it allows you to learn about the aim of the treatment and its consequences, and to be convinced that the treatment being offered is the latest and the best for your type of cancer. Getting a second opinion means your doctor stands a better chance of treating your cancer right *the first time*. You may not get another chance. If a second or even a third opinion confirms your original doctor's diagnosis and recommended course of treatment, you and your doctor will be comforted by knowing he was right.

There is no one style of doctoring that suits everyone. Getting a second opinion gives you the chance to meet someone more in tune with your needs. You need to get a second opinion from someone who has encountered and treated most, if not all, of the symptoms of your disease – a cancer specialist.

Marcia had undergone a successful mastectomy for breast cancer. Ten years later she noticed discoloration and some pain at the site of her operation and went to see a GP who had been her doctor for the past twelve years. At first the GP gave her antibiotic ointment, but when this failed to resolve her symptoms, he prescribed cortisone ointment and even suggested she wear a different brand of bra.

For ten months, month after month, he prescribed something new. By now she was in considerable pain, and the lesion on her chest was considerably larger.

She came to me for counselling, and I suggested she see an oncologist. For several weeks she demurred.

'If he thought I had cancer, he would have sent me to a specialist ages ago,' she said to me. 'After all, he referred me to the surgeon who operated on me in the first instance.'

Eventually, she agreed to see an oncologist. One look at her wound told him she had cancer. The blood test and CAT scan that followed quickly revealed it had not only recurred, it had spread to her liver. Within a few months of treatment with the hormone drug, Tamoxifen, her wound healed and her secondaries disappeared.

If your doctor is not a cancer specialist, it is likely that a cancer specialist will have a different diagnosis. If your doctor is an oncologist, a second opinion from another cancer specialist will probably confirm the original diagnosis — although the second doctor may not agree on the form of treatment. If this occurs, you may need to get a third opinion to decide the issue.

Getting three or four opinions does not mean that ten are better. At some point, you have to make a leap of faith and put your trust in one doctor — just as you decide to trust a pilot to get to your destination, knowing that if you hang around too long you may miss the plane.

Your doctor may believe that asking for another opinion reflects your refusal to face facts. He may be right, but it is still inappropriate for him to turn down your request or try to make you feel guilty for it. A good doctor will appreciate that it is not only your right to be fully informed, but that this may be your way of coping with your anxiety. Even the doctor who believes that 'There is nothing more to be done' has to accept that as long as you can breathe, it is your right to keep trying.

In the moments following my own diagnosis, my doctor told me it was imperative to remove my spleen 'or else it will grow so large it will rupture'. Had I listened to him, I would have undergone unnecessary surgery and ended up with an impaired immune system. Instead of accepting my original doctor's hopeless prognosis, I took my time to seek out other options. Eventually, I found a treatment that saved my life. And I still have my spleen.

Raising the issue of a second opinion with your doctor

What most people do is ask around and then, without telling their doctor, go to another doctor for a second opinion. There is nothing wrong with this approach, but it may cause embarrassment at a later stage, and I feel it is better to involve your doctor, not shut him out. He may feel defensive but don't be intimidated.

If your doctor is a GP, ask him straight out to refer you to a cancer specialist.

If your doctor is a cancer specialist, you could try using one of the following questions. Please note the words I have emphasised.

- 'Can you please ask one of your colleagues to comment on the results we have so far – *and* to say if he agrees with your treatment plan?'
- 'Can you please refer me to someone who will take a fresh look at my case?'
- 'I'm anxious that *we* are taking too long to find out what is wrong with me. Can you suggest someone else who can shed some light on this for *us*?'
- 'I would like you to keep taking care of me – but can *we* please get another opinion?'
- 'I think you're a wonderful doctor – and this not a rejection of you – but can we please get a second opinion?'

If your doctor's response is a hostile silence or a steely glare, or if he says something like, 'The results of your tests are clearcut; you're only wasting your time and money getting a second opinion,' my advice to you is shop around; at a time like this you need co-operation, not confrontation. Remember that those people with fighting spirit stand a better chance of survival, whether it's on the battlefield or facing a life-threatening disease.

Remember that what appears to one doctor as terminal may appear hopeful to another, and that a second opinion may make things clearer and be the spur to bring out the hope and confidence, the fighting spirit you forgot you had.

Questions to ask the second doctor

In order to avoid bias, you should ask your second doctor all the same questions you asked your first one, with a few further ones.

☞ *Do you agree with my doctor's diagnosis?*

It is most unlikely that two oncologists would disagree about your diagnosis. What is more likely is that they will differ in their choice of treatment. I know of many people who were told by their doctor that their cancer was terminal, and after consulting an oncologist discovered that their cancer was in fact curable.

☞ *What would be your treatment plan? Why is it different from my doctor's treatment plan?*

Ask him to point out the pros and cons of each treatment plan. Comparing them will give you the chance to weigh up the short-term disadvantages against the long-term benefits.

☞ *Will the treatment rid me of my disease? What will happen down the line?*

Many more treatments offer a cure today than they did ten years ago. Moreover, many doctors have noted some successful outcomes as a result of the placebo effect. Franz Inglefinger, renowned editor of the famous *New England Journal of Medicine,* noted this point in one of his articles, saying that when a patient asks his doctor, 'Will this treatment cure me?' and the doctor replies in the affirmative – *and the patient believes him* – more often than not, the treatment will work.[5]

Some treatments will not cure a disease, but they can relieve the symptoms – often for many years. Others will cure but the side effects could last a lifetime. It is your right – not your doctor's – to choose whether you wish to endure the effects of treatment if it is not going to improve your quality of life.

☞ *What would you do if you were in my shoes?*

Think carefully before deciding to ask this. To ask a stranger such a question is to place an onerous burden on him – and it could have serious consequences. A cancer specialist would know if the side effects of having no treatment were worse than those resulting from even the most intense treatments. Knowing this, he would choose to accept rather than refuse treatment. You may not, however, share his view.

We all have the potential to rise to new challenges. If you know you have options, there is almost no limit to what you can achieve – with encouragement, the love of family and friends, a doctor who won't desert you and, most of all, the realisation that others before you have prevailed. Whatever you do, don't rush into treatment without some faith in it.

three

breaking the news

*'Knowing doesn't happen at once.
You have to grow into it.'*

ANDY SIPOWICZ ('NYPD BLUE' TV SERIES)

There can be few tasks in life more difficult than breaking bad news. Most people try to get it over with as soon as possible, and there are few instances in which the person receiving the news is emotionally prepared to receive it. Unfortunately, many people choose the easy way out, say nothing, and hope someone else will do the job for them. The problem with this approach is that you cannot hide the news from your family and friends forever. It is better to break the news to your family while you are still able to help them come to terms with it. They have a right to know. If you don't tell them, they will find it harder to deal with their responses when they do find out, perhaps too late, as in the case of Marianne, a woman I counselled.

Marianne's father operated a plumbing business with her mother. Business was profitable, but the long hours took their toll, and her father began to experience chest pains. His doctor prescribed medication, but his condition slowly worsened until the doctor suggested he have coronary bypass surgery. Marianne had won a scholarship to an overseas university, her father did not want her to worry, so he and his wife decided not to tell their daughter until she returned home several months later. Shortly after surgery, complications set in, and Marianne's father unexpectedly died. Her mother broke the news to her in the only way possible: she called her long-distance.

Marianne has still not come to terms with her parents failing to tell her that her father was going to have surgery, and for not giving her the opportunity to choose to be close by him when he had his operation.

Some cultures avoid using the words 'death' or 'cancer', so doctors are told to say it's a 'cyst', 'blockage', or 'an infection that has to be removed' to ensure the patient will not be informed of the true nature of his condition. As Father Gregori, a Greek priest, told me, this can cause unbearable problems when someone is close to death. He related how he was often called by families to administer the Last Rites, too late.

'The problem with families denying the truth and leaving it so late to call me,' Father Gregori said, 'is that I often get caught up in heavy traffic, and arrive after the patient has died – of course, the family is distraught.'

Why your family, friends and workmates should be told

Your family, friends and workmates need to know your situation or else they cannot recognise and deal with their responses, or rearrange their priorities. Any disease – particularly a life-threatening one – affects not only you, but your whole family. You may feel that you have no right to burden them with your problems, but how can they show they care about you, express their love for you, unless you tell them? You will almost certainly need help during and after your treatment; how can you ask for help unless you tell them? There is also an issue of trust; if you do not confide in your family and friends, they are unlikely to ever fully trust *you* again – and they will feel less valued. It is most unlikely that your spouse or partner does not know about your condition, but if he or she doesn't, and your disease or treatment for it affects your lifestyle or your sex life, you may encounter suspicions of infidelity, indifference or lack of love.

To remove any doubts you have about the wisdom of telling them, consider how you would feel if someone you love and care about had been diagnosed with a life-threatening disease and didn't tell you. You would feel the same unassuaged, unresolved grief as the families of MIAs – soldiers missing in action – who don't know if or how their husband/father/son died, and don't even have the consolation of a body for burial.

Any situation that creates change requires an adjustment and a rearranging of priorities by those affected, whether at home or work. New tasks may have be assigned to family members and recruited friends. Adjustments in your workplace or in other pursuits will also have to be made, and for any number of reasons: your changed situation may affect your company's long-term plans, you may have to delegate work responsibilities, make sure your customers are secure, and re-order your arrangements with your bank or insurance company. You may have to defer or cancel holiday plans you made, advise your tennis club you will be unable to play for a while, and so on.

Keeping family, friends and workmates in the dark will also prevent you (and them) from dealing with whatever unfinished business may exist between you. For instance, you may have regrets over cruel or unkind remarks you made and now want to apologise; they may want your forgiveness for some act or omission on their part; you may want to thank them for their friendship and particular deeds they have done for you; they may want to express similar sentiments to you. Don't waste the unique opportunity presented by your illness to clear the air, and don't be put off if they say, 'Let's talk about it later, when you're better.' They may feel guilty that they might outlive you, you may feel resentful that they will; you may both feel you're tempting Fate by talking about these issues at this time. But what will you or they say years from now when you look back and say, 'If only I'd said what I wanted to say'?

Finally, the impulse to keep silent about your situation is, in any case, doomed to failure. Your family and others are bound to suspect that something is amiss if you are at home (but haven't retired), spend a lot of time in bed, frequently take time off work, and if your appearance changes (you lose weight, your hair falls out, you look pale and tired). Yet, if you don't open up the topic, it's hard for them to do so; they will have the distress of knowing something is wrong without the comfort of being able to help.

The futility of trying to protect someone you love from the pain of knowing the truth is revealed in Alan's story.

Alan had been operated on for pancreatic cancer. His family were concerned at his emotional strength, believed he would be unable to cope with the news, and convinced the doctor to say that he had a 'blockage', but an unrelated event which occurred while he was recuperating at home made him realise the truth. For many years his wife, obsessed with keeping a tidy kitchen, badgered him to screw the cap back on the tomato sauce bottle and return it to the pantry. Over time, he retaliated by teasingly leaving it out on purpose. Recuperating at home after surgery, he made himself a sandwich one day while his wife was out shopping and, without intent, left the bottle on the table. When she came home with all the groceries, he watched in amazement as, without a word, she screwed on the cap and put the bottle in the pantry. As soon as Alan asked her why, she burst into tears and told him the truth.

If your past pattern was to protect everyone, now is the time for you and your family to learn new and more effective ways of coping. This is not the time to shield each other from feeling and expressing emotions, but rather to drop your masks, be honest with each other, express your fears and hopes, let the love that exists between you and your family flow uninterruptedly. Your family, no less than you, needs honesty and information in order to cope.

How to break the news to family and friends

Recall how your doctor presented you with your diagnosis, and you will have some idea of how the people you tell will react when you tell them that you have a potentially life-shortening disease.

They may know you have been having tests, look unwell, and have been visiting your doctor, yet still react with shock, numbness and disbelief. They may not comprehend what you tell them – especially if you have been a well person in the past.

The time to tell them is as soon after the diagnosis has been confirmed as possible. Leave it too late and you could find yourself having to make excuses as to why you delayed.

The most insensitive and inappropriate way to break the news is to blurt out, 'I have cancer.' You will also make matters worse if you choose the wrong time and the wrong place: your wife is late for work and rushing out the door, your husband has just walked in after a hard day's work complaining of a splitting headache, your children are in the middle of doing their homework, everyone is watching 'The Simpsons'.

The most considerate way you can handle this delicate situation is to choose the right time and the right place, give a preamble to alert your family and friends you have something significant to say, then tell them what is wrong, clearly naming your cancer. Make sure at this point to impress on them that it is treatable. Pause to let this sink in, for them to ask questions, or to remain silent. Then, suggest some normal activity to stabilise the situation. In this way, you will retain your rightful role in the family, show them you intend to maintain control over all decisions affecting you.

Make sure you remember exactly what your doctor told you about treatment and its cure potential. Remind yourself that all cancers are treatable even if the prognosis is grim, so cushion the blow you are about to deliver by always adding the words, '...*and it is treatable.*' In this way, you convey a hope that there are positive things to be done.

The most direct way you can break the news is to say, 'I think you should be prepared for what I have to tell you.' Then pause, and wait for them to ask you what's wrong. Whatever you say, they will be shocked, and may say nothing as the impact of your words sinks in. This is not the time for you to keep on talking, or to ask straightaway, 'Well, what do you think?' They need time to gather their thoughts. If they don't ask you any questions or make any comment, it may be because they are frozen in their tracks and simply don't know what to say. Seconds may go by, you may be tempted to break the silence as you try to overcome your anxiety, but wait for the right moment, then tell them how *you* feel about the news, pause, then add, 'I've been to the doctor and he says that I have [whatever cancer it is] – and he thinks he can make me well. I'm going to do my best to get well.'

Another way is to say, 'You know I haven't been feeling well for some time, so I went to the doctor. The news isn't good, I'm afraid.' Pause, then say, 'According to him I have [whatever cancer it is] – *and it is treatable.*' Again, wait.

Don't expect people to respond predictably. You may be pleasantly surprised; you could be sadly disappointed. They may rush out of the room, throw themselves into your arms, swear volubly, or even faint. At this point, perhaps the wisest thing you can say is, 'Why don't I put on the kettle and make us all a cup of tea? Then we'll talk.'

It is important that you handle this delicate situation properly. You need to give them the chance to react in their own way, and at the same time show you intend to maintain control over all decisions affecting you.

Bear in mind that the ages, disposition and levels of understanding of family members and friends will vary, so it may be advisable to break the news separately to each of them. I will discuss the issue of telling children further on, but in general, keep it simple to begin with and emphasise your willingness to answer questions, now or later.

It may seem contrived, but the technique of 'mirroring' (see Chapter 2) will help ensure they understand what you have told them. Get them to repeat what you have said, and ask them, perhaps a few times, if they have any questions. You may want to share as much as you know with them, but use your discretion, and keep checking to make sure they really do understand. And listen. The only way you will have any idea of what they are thinking, feeling, and fearing is to listen, and then respond appropriately.

Telling older parents

Protecting those around you from the news can be tiring and futile; in the case of older parents it can be unnecessarily cruel. What happened to me is a case in point.

At the time of my first cancer diagnosis, my elderly father had lived with us for almost thirteen years. I was his only child and my relationship with him was extremely close; we kept no secrets from each other. My wife insisted that we withhold the news from him on account of his age and his heart condition, and I was still too numb with the news of my diagnosis, and much too tired from my condition, to contest her wishes. As the weeks went by, my skin colour changed to yellow from carrot juice, and I lost considerable amount of weight. I could not look him in the eye, and felt guilty every time my wife and I talked behind closed doors.

Eventually, I decided to tell him, whereupon he heaved a sigh of relief and told me that my appearance had already alerted him to the fact that I was gravely ill, and that he had spent sleepless nights worrying about me. From the moment I told him all about my condition and why I was using alternative programs to try and cure myself, he helped me prepare the numerous juices required by them, and was a constant source of encouragement. Without his help, I would never have had the time or energy to undertake, let alone maintain, my strict alternative regimens.

There can be no valid reason for not telling your parents, unless they are totally incapable of understanding anything. You may believe you will be sparing them pain and suffering by withholding the news from them, but there is a greater probability that your eventual 'unexpected' death will cause them even greater shock and mental disturbance – more so when they realise that you knew all along and didn't trust them enough to tell them.

You can help ease their pain by giving them the chance to come to terms with their anticipatory grief while you are still alive. It will most certainly give all of you the opportunity to resolve past differences, express feelings you've been reluctant or afraid to express, and forge new bonds of love, friendship and affection. As with me, giving your aged parents the opportunity to help you as they did when you were a child may give them a new lease of life, as poignant as the situation is likely to be for them.

Breaking the news to children
WHY CHILDREN SHOULD BE TOLD

Your first response to a cancer diagnosis may be, 'Don't tell the children.' You may say, 'Let kids be kids', thinking that they will have enough to worry about when they're older, or that they're too young to understand. It is vital you remind yourself that every child is a person, an individual with feelings. You cannot override children's emotions in the belief you are protecting them without paying a price.

Children have the longest ears in the world. They will find out one way or another, sooner or later; it is far better that they find out from you. Imagine your young daughter overhearing someone say, 'He only has a fifty-fifty chance,' and, in her innocence, asking either you or someone else, 'What's a fifty-fifty chance?' No matter how determined you may have been not to say anything, you will now have no choice but to tell. Or picture the situation where your child is confronted by a teacher or a friend who says, 'I am so sorry to hear about your poor dear father.'

If your child finds out you are ill from someone else, they may feel that they are unimportant; something serious has happened in their own family, yet no one bothered to tell them they are likely to feel marginalised and unimportant – and they will feel the tension between their innate sense that something is wrong (and young children always know!) and your silence. When their instincts tell them one thing and you tell them another – or even nothing – they will assume their instincts are wrong. You diminish the survival mechanism of children when you teach them, directly or indirectly, that instinct is not to be trusted. If, as a parent, you don't teach your children trust, who will? Moreover, how can they trust *you* if you're not prepared to trust them? This can have potentially serious consequences. I know. This is what happened to me.

In her belief that she was protecting our children, my wife insisted that we did not tell them about my disease. Later, and against her wishes, I did tell them, and tried to explain why I had failed to do so sooner. I was fairly certain they had accepted my explanation, but over the subsequent years, my once-close relationship with one of my sons broke down, and I was at a loss to explain why. Many years later, I discovered that the cause of his anger, and our inability to communicate with each other, was *because I had failed to take him into my confidence*. Although my wife was convinced that she had successfully hidden the news about my condition from him, he said he had known all along.

Children also have long antennae, and are particularly sensitive to changing vibrations in the home: they notice when the rhythm of life is altered, when you are unwell, when your thoughts are elsewhere. Putting on a brave front when you are fearful won't fool them, especially if they notice that you're continually tired, are seeing your doctor frequently, and are concerned with problems you previously ignored. They are also sensitive to silences. They will feel that something is wrong if every time they come within earshot you stop talking, or if they see you or your wife or husband whispering with your doctor as he is about to leave your house. If you fail to tell them what's happening, they may suspect the truth or come to the wrong conclusion about your behaviour. They may assume that they have done something wrong.

Your treatment program may require that you spend some time in hospital; if your children don't understand why you 'have to go away', and if you don't return, they will probably end up having to face every child's greatest fear: abandonment. The saying, 'Children are good observers and poor interpreters,' was never more apt than at a time like this. If, for example, they knew a grandparent had died in hospital and your wife tells them that you have to go to hospital, it is not unnatural for them to assume you are going to hospital to die.

As I will explain later in this chapter, it is vital you know what your children understand about death *before* you break the news – even if your cancer can be cured. Children often fantasise, and may think they did something to make you ill, and now are to blame. For instance, your daughter or son may think, 'Dad asked me to walk the dog, and I didn't. Now he's ill. Maybe it's my fault.' If you don't or can't tell them, and you then die, they may assume you left them because of something they did or didn't do and so will carry unnecessary guilt throughout their lives. You run the risk of adding anger to their guilt – an unnecessary legacy – if they feel there was something they could have done to help and you denied them the opportunity. Family members and friends can show great insensitivity, can hurt the feelings of your children and increase their guilt burden when they link their behaviour to your condition, especially in a younger child, and say, for example, 'Your mother's ill. Don't upset her more.'

Your children should always share your sense of hope, but they will cope better if you are realistic and acknowledge that although you will fight for survival, death is inevitable – it will come, sooner or later.

They will admire your courage if you prevail against the odds, and if you don't, will know you gave it your best shot, courageously and responsibly. The most admired heroes or heroines are not necessarily those who prevail against overwhelming forces, but those who do not shrink from the battle. In the fact of this, there can be few greater legacies to leave your children than the knowledge that you were a hero or a heroine in your life – and that you didn't abandon them on purpose.

Dealing with grief needs to start while people are still alive, so don't withdraw in the hope they will find it easier when you die. Your continuing presence and making yourself available at all times, if possible, will help to restore equilibrium, and show everyone the wisdom of the Buddha that life can be found only by living in the present moment. Seeing you face your disease can help them grow in their ability to face other tough experiences in their lives, become more responsible about themselves, and develop self-confidence and independence. They're also more likely to become sensitive to the needs of others, and mature in their ability to love and understand someone other than themselves.

A number of studies have shown that people see renewed relationships, especially with their children, as one of the most positive outcomes of their illness.[1] Painful as it may be for them to see you suffer, a long illness can prepare them to cope with your death, whenever it may be, far better than if you died suddenly.

WHY YOU SHOULD DO THE TELLING

At the best of times, talking to children can present difficulties in communication. We forget how we communicated (or failed to communicate) with our parents, now talk about the 'generation gap', and when we try to be 'with it', are told we're 'uncool'. You could be daunted by the prospect, but you have no choice. You have to talk.

There are many people who believe parents are not qualified or trained to deal with the sensitivities of children, and that they should call upon an expert – even a doctor – to handle the matter. There are eight reasons why I disagree with this view:

1   The ways in which people (and children *are* people!) respond to a life-threatening situation are a natural part of life and not symptoms of some underlying disease requiring medical intervention.
2   You are the parent: no one knows your children better than you, your spouse or partner.
3   *You* have to live with your children. Someone else may be extremely qualified, but they don't have to live with the consequences of their remarks.
4   Your children's way of thinking and their view of the world is largely influenced by you; they tend to see life through your eyes. You are their role model, for good or bad.
5   Doctors are not always the most skilled communicators.

6   Delegating the task to someone else denies you and your child the opportunity to face each other's pain, to comfort each other – and for them to ask questions.

7   They may think you handed the matter of telling to someone else because you don't want them to know what you know.

8   Asking someone else to tell your children is the clearest indicator of your inability to face reality at the same time you expect them to.

By all means get advice if you feel unsure about the facts, but don't pass the buck. Readjusting to a new situation requires time, patience and understanding. As long as you are honest, patient, loving and available to them, as long as you tell them how much you care, you will be amazed at how well your children will come through this difficult time.[2]

WHEN AND HOW MUCH TO TELL

As a parent, you undoubtedly feel responsible for your children, that it is your duty to protect them from fear, worry and uncertainty. You are not alone in believing this, or that you should put off telling your children until you feel 'the time is right', but these views are unrealistic.

You have to break the news as soon as possible after your diagnosis has been confirmed, even to your younger children. Explain the purpose of the treatment, while you are being treated, and how you are being treated. Tell them about the side effects, and tell them when you are starting new treatments. Tell them only as much as they can understand. As long as you bear these points in mind, you should find it easier and easier to speak to them as time goes by. If they don't ask you any questions or make any comment, they could be frozen with shock, simply don't know what to say, so allow them to react in their own time, in their own way.

How and what you tell them will determine the way they cope, now and in the future, so before talking to them, decide beforehand *what* you are going to say, then decide *how* to say it in as clear, concise and gentle a way as possible. Choose your words carefully so you don't unduly alarm them. Pick the right time and place, tell them separately if there is a clear difference in their ages, and remember, everyone will respond differently. Don't blurt out that you have cancer, rather lead them to it by telling them how you have been feeling, that you've been to the doctor, that you're sad but optimistic, and pause between sentences. Don't tell them while they're doing their homework, watching TV or racing off to play with their friends. Choose the familiarity of their or your bedroom in which to break the news and remember, it's important that you communicate your feelings as well as the facts. Leave plenty of time between sentences for them to gather their thoughts or ask questions. If your children have been of assistance to you and your spouse, tell them — and don't let them forget that you love them. Remember that what you say, and the tone of voice in which you say it, will leave a lasting impression.

Whatever you do, don't forget to advise their teachers of your condition as soon as possible, so they can be prepared to deal with any problems when and if they arise.

MAKING SURE THEY UNDERSTAND

Keep your message simple to begin with. No matter how you try to cushion the impact of the news, the shock will shut down their senses so they will hear little or nothing. As they become less numb, they are likely to read more (or less) into your words than you intended, so it is vital that you check with them to find out what they understood.

Children use their imagination to fill in the gaps, so try hard not to leave out anything important, or else they could distort what you have told them. Don't underestimate the ability of your handicapped child to understand, or think that his or her emotions will be less affected. I have a mentally disabled stepson who continually amazes us with his insights and awareness of what's happening.

The best way to check is to ask them directly, 'Do you understand what I am telling you?' Listen attentively. They may ask you to repeat what you have said, not because they are unintelligent, but because they require constant reassurance that they have understood you. Whatever you do, don't be evasive. Answer their questions as simply as possible, and answer them whenever they ask. Don't say, 'I'll tell you later.' Keep checking to make sure they understand. It's important for them to talk, so don't close the door to your room – or your heart.

Don't overload them with details – you could end up saying things that are best left for a time when everyone is calmer. You will alarm and confuse them if you overdo the scientific information, or give frightening and extensive details of your disease. Unless your lifestyle is going to change dramatically (such as no longer being able to afford to keep them at private school), don't burden them with more problems than they can manage. In particular, don't trouble them about your financial situation, as this will add to their insecurity.

There's also no need for them to suffer anxiety waiting for your test results, so if they're old enough to understand, let them share in your disappointment, or your joy, *after* you know. Keeping them informed on an ongoing basis after your treatment will save them imagining a situation far worse than the reality. For example, if you fail to tell them that the therapy you are about to undergo may cause you to lose your hair and you suddenly start wearing a wig or a hat, they will get a shock. You'll go a long way towards maintaining their trust and help offset their sense of alienation if they feel they can always ask you questions whenever they want to. Once you've told them, continue to include them in all future family discussions so they aren't left alone with their fears, can share the responsibilities that may arise, and don't feel abandoned.

EXAMPLES OF HOW TO TELL

Remind yourself that telling children you have cancer has to satisfy *their* curiosity and allay *their* fears, not yours. You may be surprised at the responses of your children, no matter how well you think you know them; children often teach us more than we teach them, as Anna discovered when she came to me for counselling after she was diagnosed with leiomyosarcoma, a rare form of cancer.

Anna was anxious how her children, aged between six and thirteen, would react to her telling them about her cancer, particularly six-year-old Marylou. I suggested she tell them straight out, but separately. When she told Marylou, the response was beyond her wildest expectations.

ANNA: You know I've been in hospital. What I didn't tell you
  is that I am ill with cancer.

MARYLOU: Are you going to die?
ANNA: We all have to die, darling. But I hope I don't have to
for a long time.
MARYLOU: Don't worry, Mum. I love you like elastic. No
matter where you go, it will stretch.

For your and your children's sake, it is essential that you retain a sense of optimism. Keep reminding yourself that cancer is a word, not a sentence. Even so, don't shirk your responsibility of telling the truth.

- ☞ 'I am going to do my best to get better. I may not succeed, but I will try.'
- ☞ 'Daddy is sick with something that some people die from – but the doctor thinks he can make him well. I hope so, too.'

You may be encouraged by their response if you can show determination and a will to live. When I told my sons about my first cancer, they were aged fourteen, sixteen and eighteen. I told them the reason I had been off work for some time was because I had a rare form of leukemia, and in the same breath added, 'But I am going to beat it, even though the doctors don't think I can.' They were at once shocked, saddened, reduced to tears, and enthusiastic about my attitude. Their united response was, 'What can we do to help you, Dad?'

Key considerations before and after breaking the news

What do you do when the dust has settled and they've caught their breath? In a time of great uncertainty, it is vital you know what to expect and what to do. You can ease your children's fears if you endeavour to answer all their questions, bearing in mind their differing ages and levels of understanding. There may be many questions you are unable to answer, but if you acknowledge this, show you have nothing to hide, and are willing to share what you know, you will help your children feel more comfortable with *their* uncertainty.

You will help them lift the veil of uncertainty by relating the answers as you find them. If you explain why you look and feel the way you do, and if you do so with confidence, the chances are that your children will accept these changes more easily.

Many parents mistakenly burden their children with adult respon-sibilities when they say, for example, 'You're a man now. If you cry, you'll only upset your mother.' Or, 'You're the mum now. It's up to you to take care of your little sister.' To offset the change in emotional climate in your home, as well as your own physical changes, try to keep things as normal as possible by maintaining a daily routine involving everyone. Filling your and their appropriate roles will help remind your children that you are still a family, and will help to ensure continuity of duties, obligations and pastimes: doing their homework, taking out the garbage, raking the leaves, feeding the dog, watching TV. Children often cope better than adults, provided they are kept informed and busy, and are given the support of a lov-ing family. And remember to keep handing out their pocket money!

This is also not the time to send them packing to a distant aunt or cousin – a not uncommon occurrence following the death of a parent. This will not only prevent them from helping out, but will disrupt their routine, and could result in banishing them to emotional exile, making it hard for them to maintain trusting, secure relationships. This is what happened to Sophie, a woman in her mid-forties who came to me for counselling following a diagnosis of breast cancer.

Some years earlier, Sophie had been in therapy in an attempt to sort out her failed marriage and to find out why, as soon as she thought she had found her ideal new partner among her many suit-ors, he left her. When Sophie was nine, her father told her that her mother had 'gone far away', refused to tell her until she was sixteen that her mother had died. Fearing further abandonment, Sophie had became dependent, a 'hanger-on', always childlike, traits that initially appealed but later irritated her husband and subsequent boyfriends. Her pain eased when, through therapy, she recognised what had hap-pened to her, learned to show more independence, and was eventu-ally able to make a lasting relationship.

In many cases, the result can be a lifelong feeling of inadequacy or guilt – children feel that their parent didn't love them enough to live, or that they were in some way responsible for their parent's ill-ness or death. They could, in later years, find gaps in their reminis-cences about you, and may resent your spouse or partner for failing to keep them within the family circle. Don't send your children away, physically or emotionally. Your disease is more than enough for them to cope with, and how will you rescue them later?

The side effects of your treatment can be distressing to younger children, so you may find it necessary to ask for help. Bear in mind that adding another person to the household can seem like an invasion of their territory, and make them feel that things are far worse than they really are. If you do need help, perhaps because you are a single parent, it is essential you call the same person every time, to keep change to a minimum.

You will almost certainly become the topic of conversation among the children in the neighbourhood, and this can prove difficult for your children, especially if they don't want to admit that anything has changed at home. It is important that you let them know you are willing to talk to their friends, and to show them you are normal. In this way, you have a unique opportunity to educate them about cancer, and show them how it can bring family and friends even closer.

With the focus of the household shifted towards you, your children may start to 'act up' to gain attention. You may think that this is not the time to maintain or enforce discipline, but it is essential that you do. Children feel safe, secure and less vulnerable within known limits. You need to reassure them that you understand how they might be feeling at this time, but that you will not condone bad behaviour. Expressing your love and acceptance of their feelings will go a long way towards obtaining acceptance of yours.

Facing the unknown as a family unit is less threatening for everyone, and if you share activities you will get to spend more time together. Look to take part in activities that do not tire you, and which involve creative pursuits that can help your children express their frustration and their anger, and overcome their sadness and depression. If you are not well enough or feel ill-equipped to engage in therapeutic child's play, such as sand-play or drawing, ask your doctor to refer you to a children's psychologist. Teaching your children how to express themselves creatively in this time of crisis can help them discover new ways to deal with their problems now and in later life.

This is not the time to hide your feelings, however sad you may be about the effect of your disease on your children. Letting them see how you feel, will help them recognise that it's acceptable to honour their feelings rather than suppress them, bring you closer, and relieve the fear and pain of losing you. If you feel your emotions are out of control and are concerned about the effect of this on your children, talk to your doctor. He may prescribe a short course of anti-depressants, or refer you to a psychiatrist or counsellor to help you get a grip on things.

Facing the unknown with others can provide additional comfort, so reach out to your extended family and friends, especially those with children of similar ages to your own. Joining a support group can also be of immense benefit, more so if other members have children or grandchildren of the same age. Your children will feel consoled by meeting other children in a similar situation.

WHAT TO DO WHEN THEY ASK, 'ARE YOU GOING TO DIE?' In our society, topics such as cancer and death are pushed aside, or papered over with euphemisms. Talking about these issues to children is made even harder because of their age and the perceived need to protect them from reality but, as many authorities have shown, reality catches up, often with disastrous consequences in later life.[3]

The issue of death may not be one you wish to entertain, but it is likely to pop into your children's minds the moment you mention the word 'cancer' or if one of their friends asks, 'Is your Mum (or Dad) going to die?'

So ask yourself what experience of illness or death have they had in the past, how was it explained to them and, most importantly, how well did they understand it? Look for clues. For instance, your son's pet dog may have been run over or put down because it had a serious disease; their grandfather or someone close to them may have died; they may have found a dead bird in the garden. You might consider them too young to talk to about disease and death (and maybe they are), but remember, death and dying are the stuff of television news bulletins, dramas and sitcoms. In almost every cartoon someone gets killed, maimed, brained, or dismembered – and then reappears intact in the next program. No news report is complete without its mandatory sequence of natural disasters, random slaying, mob violence and military precision killings. It would be the rare child who has not heard the words 'disease', 'heart attack', 'cancer', 'death' and 'dying' and, depending on age, each one will attach a different meaning to each of these words, so it is important you know what they know before you talk to them.

If possible, draw this information out of them over a few days in order to gauge their level of understanding *before* you break the news. To do so, ask them what they think words such as cancer, disease, sickness or death mean. Obviously, you don't want to alarm them; a child's mind processes information differently and at different ages, so don't generalise or make assumptions about what *you* think they know. On another occasion, ask them if they're worried about you, and why. You stand a better chance of correcting any misinformation they may have while everything still appears normal.

Children are sensitive to our moods, so if you are defensive and unwilling to discuss cancer or death realistically, the message they will receive is that you believe these subjects are taboo; whereas if you confront your disease in an open and honest way, your words and actions will be a source of strength and comfort for them in facing future grief and loss. It's a fact of life that in order to grow and mature, everyone – no matter how old – needs to experience disappointment, sadness and loss. Conversely, you will surely weaken your children's coping capacity if you try to shield them from emotional pain and grief by telling them 'kind lies'.

There are many excellent books that deal in great detail with this complex issue, and I have listed a few of them in the footnotes to this chapter.[4] As an introduction to them, and to help you feel more at ease about breaking the news about your illness to your children in the most appropriate way, I will highlight some of the key elements you should be aware of, especially if you believe your child is too young to understand.

As you read through them, bear in mind that many characteristics overlap, and that while there are definite stages, children advance or regress through them at their own pace. Psychologists concur that, for children, death is a complex, ever-changing kaleidoscope of mutually contradictory paradoxes that vary from person to person, and from culture to culture.[5]

UP TO TWO YEARS OLD

Experts working with children are often surprised by how much children *do* understand; babies of six to eighteen months have been observed showing signs of sorrow. Even the youngest of children can sense when their routine is changed, although the younger they are, the less they will understand *why* things are different.

Until the age of two, any form of separation will cause anxiety; but the more secure a child feels about his own sense of self, the less fearful he will be of separation. In this regard, it has been suggested that the game of Peek-a-Boo (from the Old English words meaning 'Alive or dead?') may not be only a simple nursery game, but a vital factor in the establishment of an independent individual. If you have ever played this game with a child, even as young as three months old, you will know that as long as you keep your face covered – i.e. seem absent – they will be distressed, but as soon as you uncover your face, they are comforted and smile with relief.

The interest shown by young children in disappearance and return may indeed be their first experience with non-being or death. Even at this age children gradually come to realise that many things do not return – as when, for instance, they say, 'All gone.'

FROM TWO TO SIX

From about the age of two until they are about five or six, children develop confidence and trust by the reassurance of your return, whether from the shops or from work. However, if their favourite dog or cat was killed, they will almost certainly come to realise that loss sometimes means no return.

Some psychologists believe that children between three and five have no knowledge of death, and that the realisation of the inevitability of it does not occur until they are nine or ten. They may not be mature enough to have the concept of death, but there is undeniably a felt sense of loss. The inexpressible grief accompanying the death of a pet is indelible – people who are asked to recall their first experience of death invariably say it was the loss of a pet.

It is important you bear this in mind. If, in response to the question of where the dead pet or person has gone, the answer you give is 'heaven' or 'somewhere far away', these terms will become associated with permanent loss rather than providing the reassurance you intended. At this age children are not quite able to grasp concepts such as time, death and nothingness, so it may be some considerable time before they accept that their pet or their grandfather is not coming back.

In the face of this, it is worth noting children in this age group see death as reversible. Their favourite cartoon characters are killed but come back to life, often within the same television program. They make the same assumption about people when they are told they have died.

Children at this stage cannot imagine a world without their parents.[6] They will only discover a sense of self when they realise they can survive without their parents, and are quite distinct from them. In other words, it is only when children recognise separateness that they are able to understand the finality of death.

FROM SIX TO NINE

From about five or six to about nine, awareness of death may be experienced in various ways. The fairy tales you told your children when they were younger may now have progressed into stories where the hero, for instance, slays a dragon or kills the villain. At this time, they develop an adult view of death. Refusing to answer questions about death, regarding the subject as taboo, and allowing them attend funerals without adequate explanations of what is happening, can create a lifelong, morbid fascination with death.

Young children who are allowed to watch violent movies, and that includes news bulletins, see death as 'not alive', and almost always the result of doing bad deeds. It will also almost always be associated with punishment for bad behaviour where death (the potential and reality of loss) is invoked through the bogeyman who 'comes to take naughty children away'. Not surprisingly, many children become naughty in an attempt to prove their 'aliveness' and deny the potential of death.

Most children in this age group will come to realise that death is final, others will still believe that dead people come back to life.

Boys, especially, need to know that it's not 'unmanly' to cry, that feeling bad, frightened and angry are normal emotions. It will help them enormously if you remind them you also experience such moods.

Children at this age are also fascinated by ghosts and magic. It is during this period of development that children, no doubt influenced by these stories, come to imagine that they can also influence events in the world. For example, you may have sent your child to the bedroom as punishment for bad behaviour. Alone in their room and raging at your actions, they may express the wish that you were dead. If, at some later stage, you either die or tell them that you may die, they may feel responsible and guilty for what has happened. If you do become sick after you have said something like 'You make me sick' or 'I'm getting sick and tired of telling you to put your clothes away,' your child is almost certainly going to feel responsible for your condition. It is essential to reassure them that they are in no way responsible for your disease.

FROM NINE TO TWELVE

Between about nine and twelve, the feelings of your children will not be vastly different from your own. By now they will have made the transition from seeing death as a person (the bogeyman) or an object separate from themselves to seeing death as a part of life – including their own.

Children at this time are fascinated by the biology of death, entranced by ghost stories, ready to dissect insects, frogs and lizards. On the other hand, they will bond with their pet as part of the family and, should it die, will want a proper burial for it.

Their notion of what is living and not-living is usually well defined by this age. Abandonment and separation will still loom large in their thoughts, so they will be affected by anything they feel challenges their security, and are likely to imagine situations far worse than they might experience in reality. In the face of this, it is essential you are open and honest with them, bearing in mind that the most comforting reassurance you can always give them is that you or someone else – your spouse or partner, parent or godparent – will always be there for them.

TEENAGERS

In general, children are more afraid of separation and loss than death itself until they become teenagers; then their sense of self matures, and they develop a greater sense of what their own death may mean.

Just as younger children may become naughty in order to deny death, so teenagers, even adults, often engage in dangerous and death-defying activities to assert their 'alive-ness'. What is regarded by many people as the age of fearlessness may, in fact, be a time of great fear. This attitude is largely unconscious since, with their belief that they have a lifetime ahead of them, most teenagers view themselves as immortal.

For these reasons, paradoxical as it may seem, teenagers may find it more difficult than younger children to believe or accept that you have a life-threatening disease. Don't assume that because they're older they can deal with all their problems. This is a difficult time for them, but if you can find the time to share your feelings with your teenage son or daughter, you will help them immeasurably in overcoming their grief.

Teenagers rarely show their grief verbally; they displace it onto external situations and activities such as poor schoolwork, truancy, stealing, daydreaming. They may get depressed, become overly aggressive, withdrawn or even stop talking. And don't be fooled if they assume an outward air of toughness. Faced with what they may believe is your inevitable death, their attitude may be 'What's the use?'.

With teenagers, as with adults, you cannot predict how anyone will respond. Remember, expect the unexpected.

THE QUESTION OF DEATH

A woman came to Buddha with her dead son in her arms and pleaded with him to bring her son back to life.

The Buddha told her that if she could collect a mustard seed from a household in which no one had ever died, he would grant her wish.

In desperation she went from house to house, from village to village, until several days later, wearied by her efforts, she came to the Buddha and said, 'There is no house where there has been no death or one where there has been no grief.'

So saying, she came to realise that death comes to everyone.

When children come straight out and ask, 'What is death?', 'Are you going to die?' and 'Am I going to die?' you have to answer them as truthfully and as matter-of-factly as possible without hurrying them through the subject. You owe it to them to be as open and as honest as possible. Remind yourself that if you can share what you feel and believe, you will make it easier for them to cope – not only with your disease, but with any other life crisis they will surely encounter at some later stage in their lives. If you deny the reality of death, so will they.

If you feel uncomfortable with the answer you're giving to some question, or simply do not know what to say, then all you have to say is, 'I don't know.' The following excerpt from Doris Buchanan Smith's sensitively written book, *A Taste of Blackberries,* highlights how easy it is to provide an honest answer, and how children see through lies.

A little boy, whose friend had died from a bee sting, asked his neighbour, Mrs Mullins, 'Why did Jamie have to die?'

The question lay in the air between us. The sound of it shocked me, but Mrs Mullins didn't act surprised.

'Honey, one of the hardest things you have to learn is that some questions do not have answers.' I nodded. This made more sense than if she tried to sell me some junk about God meeting angels.

'What's it like to be dead? Or is that another one of those questions?'

'It's one of those questions,' she said. 'You just don't know until you can find out yourself, and apparently you can't come back and tell what you found out.'[7]

Children are remarkably able to deal with reality, so satisfying their curiosity by giving them a biological explanation of what death means may make it easier to explain what happens after life. You may feel more comfortable presenting your children with half-truths and fantastic ideas, but if they later find out you were wrong or arrive at a different interpretation, they may be shocked to discover you don't know everything. As a parent, you have a unique opportunity to help your child's psychological growth by respecting their efforts to figure out the meaning of death without thrusting your interpretation of it onto them.

As I said earlier, you can use the experience of a pet's death to explain that being dead means that the body:

— has stopped working and won't do the things it used to do;

—·can't be fixed, can't start again;

— won't see, hear, smell, walk, talk or think;
— can't feel hot or cold, happy or sad,
— can't feel any more pain.

Your particular religion may provide you with clues on what to say. Call on the services of your priest, rabbi or teacher to recommend a suitable book, or ask your librarian to suggest one appropriate to your child's age, as a follow-up to your discussion, not a substitute. As psychologist Dr Alice Miller points out, *the key to communicating with a child is to provide an answer that satisfies the child, not the parent.*[8]

There are many words and expressions you should avoid because of their implications at a later stage; words and phrases such as 'passed away', 'left us', 'gone on', 'gone far away', 'gone on a long journey', or 'gone to heaven'.

The risk of misinterpretation by young children is obvious. If, for example, at some later date, you choose to take a holiday, your children may think you will not return. Avoid the word 'heaven', in particular, unless you can explain, with conviction, what the word means and know that your child understands it *to the same extent*. 'Forever' has no meaning to a young child who measures his life by such distant events as birthdays, Christmas, and the start of a new term at school. As for the word 'sleep', I wonder how many adults are insomniacs because they still associate the word 'sleep' with 'death'?

Age and death are usually connected in a child's mind, so if they ask, 'Are you going to die?' the most honest answer you can give is to say, 'I don't know.' If your prognosis is not grim, you could add, 'Everyone dies some time, but I don't expect to die until you are very old and have children of your own. Sometimes people get very sick or have a bad accident and die before they're very, very old. Most of the time, people don't die until they're very, very, *very* old.' [9]

Don't impose on your children the notion that death is linked to revenge or punishment, and don't present them with a fanciful doctrine they will later need to unlearn. If you want them to go through life with as little fear of death as possible and be able to deal with anything life throws at them, I believe the most valuable legacy you can bequeath them is to show them that death is a natural event, not something to be feared.

SAYING GOODBYE

Whether they think it or say it, the thoughts uppermost in your children's minds are bound to be 'What will happen to me?', 'Who will take care of me when you go to hospital?' and 'Will we still live in the same house?' To help them overcome their anxiety and reassure them, you need to make them understand that they will not be left alone.

Abandonment and rejection – even the threat of them – are the greatest fears of a child. As long as you communicate that you are neither rejecting nor abandoning them, that your eventual and possible departure is not of your own choice, and they did nothing wrong, you may render your parting a 'sweet sorrow' rather than a wrenching life-enduring tragedy. To that end, when the time eventually comes for you to die, it is important to actually say, 'Goodbye'. Certainly, it is hard to say, but *not* saying it will carry a more painful and lasting legacy

In answer to the big question, 'Where will you go when you die?' tell them, 'Into your memory.' And when they ask, 'But what happens if I forget to think about you?' say, 'Don't worry. I'll remind you.'

four

the right doctoring

'The secret of the care of the patient is in
caring for the patient.'

Dr Francis Weld Peabody

Who is the right doctor for you?

Before deciding which treatment is best for your cancer, you need to
find the right doctor. But who is the right doctor for you? Is it the
doctor who saves your life or the one who gives you hope? Is it the
one who diagnoses your problem right the first time or the one who
doesn't make you feel rushed? Is it the one who explains everything
to you in a comforting way or the one who makes all your decisions
for you?

Most people equate the right doctor with the right treatment on
the basis of the **result** of the treatment. If the treatment doesn't work,
no matter how friendly and attentive he may have been, the doctor is
seen as a failure. If the treatment is successful the doctor, no matter
how abrupt or unfriendly he may have been, is regarded as 'the best'.

You need the right doctor *and* you need the right treatment. The
two are not always found together, but when they are, you stand a
better chance of winning.

The right balance: care and cure

In spite of advances in neurology and psychology confirming the
relationship of mind and body, many in the medical profession prefer
to remain focused on biology and chemistry, manipulating tissues
and cells to treat diseases, rather than seeing how beliefs and feelings
can influence physical states. We need doctors who balance technology with psychology, pharmacology with philosophy, and the results

of blood tests and X-rays with your character, your fears and your expectations. This may appear to be a fanciful wish, but *in the face of a life-threatening disease, we want to be cared for as much as we want to be cured*.

Science has, indeed, produced some dramatic results. The extent to which sanitation, personal and food hygiene, improved nutrition, pre- and post-natal care and vaccination have prolonged and saved untold millions of lives convinced doctors that science, in whatever form, would eventually rid mankind of all diseases. Advances in anaesthesia and surgical technology allow limbs to be sewn back, arteries and organs replaced, and cancers removed. Pharmacological weapons — insulin, antibiotics, and a host of cancer and cardiac drugs — have been developed. More discoveries at the genetic level hold incredible promise for the future. Yet all this technical progress has its disadvantages. The lure of science, and the often miraculous recoveries of people after being administered an antibiotic, convinced doctors that there was almost nothing they could not fix. People, too, have come to believe that most, if not all, of their illnesses can be cured by one drug or another; all you need is a prescription from your doctor. These expectations are often unrealistic. There are some diseases for which there are no cures and no medicines to treat the symptoms. There are many diseases for which there are medicines that can treat the symptoms but not cure the patient.

On top of this, specialisation has diminished the opportunity for doctors to build relationships with their patients. The doctor who cannot fathom his patient's problem invariably sends him to a specialist who may, in turn, send him to another specialist. This process may well enhance the study of that particular disease, but it totally ignores the emotions and feelings of the patient.

Doctors may believe it is the medicine they dispense that cures, but it is their mere presence that is often the best medicine. You know this yourself when, no matter how ill or distressed you are, your anxiety level is reduced and you can say, 'I feel so much better already,' as soon as he arrives to attend you.

You want a doctor who makes you feel this way — one who improves your emotional well-being, boosts your confidence and stimulates your will to live. But you also want a doctor who is an expert in cancer — *your* type of cancer.

Why you need a cancer specialist

Cancer specialists are in an unrivalled position to help you; they know from theory and practice how your disease develops, and are skilled and up-to-date in the techniques of alleviating symptoms as well as cure. Only a specialist is experienced in selecting and managing a large variety of treatments: surgery, chemotherapy, radiotherapy, gene therapy. Only a specialist can marshal the resources of other highly trained, supportive-care people: nurses, physiotherapists, nutritionists, counsellors. A cancer specialist is often qualified to perform tumor surgery. And if you look carefully, you can find specialists in whom the 'carer' and 'curer' come together, people for whom treating your symptoms is as important as caring for you as a person.

Where to go if care is lacking

In my own case, I have been fortunate to have two great specialists who shared their encyclopaedic knowledge of cancer with me, supported my taking an active role in my recoveries, and attended to me with compassion and empathy. Because such paragons are by no means the norm among specialists, many cancer patients continue to search desperately for the caring doctor, often among alternative practitioners. If you find that an alternative practitioner provides that missing element, fine – but *don't* let him dissuade you from obtaining an orthodox medical treatment that could save your life. The other thing to remember, if your cancer specialist is not meeting your psychological needs, is that you can seek help from, for example, a psychologist, a counsellor, a friend, a fellow cancer survivor. If you are severely depressed, you can consult a psychiatrist, a trained doctor who is aware of the side effects caused by some cancer treatments. You may be compelled to rely on a cancer specialist for your medical care and on others for your emotional, psychological and spiritual well-being.

Risks in not choosing a cancer specialist

If your doctor has been so insensitive as to say that there is nothing more he can do for you, it is only natural to cast around for someone else to throw you a lifeline. If the person offering to save you is not a cancer specialist, you could be exposing yourself to grave danger. You may be at even greater risk receiving treatment from an untrained doctor using proven methods improperly than from an alternative practitioner using unproven methods. (The question of alternative treatments is discussed in more detail in Chapter 7.)

Here are some points to consider in making your decision.

1   A far-reaching study on undergraduate medical education in Australia, published in 1994, showed that university lecturers in Australia and elsewhere in Europe were not well-informed about the rates of occurrence of various cancers, and had differing views about treatment goals and options.[1] This is a powerful argument in favour of seeking treatment for cancer from a cancer specialist.

2   A general practitioner may, on average, only deal with one or two cases of cancer a year – and maybe never the one you have.

3   In your current state of confusion, anxiety and fear, you are highly persuadable and can be misled, not only by sincere but inexpert practitioners, but by those who seek to make money out of the vulnerability of others. I have counselled a number of people with cancer who, for various reasons, persist in being treated by a practitioner they know is not a cancer specialist only to discover, when their condition has deteriorated, that they have run out of time, and sometimes money as well.

4   Doctors are accountable for their actions, alternative practitioners are not. You have no right of recourse if you use unregulated practitioners.

5   It is wrong to assume that all alternative practitioners will treat you more humanely and inspiringly than all conventional doctors. My own experience and those of many of the people I have counselled confirms this, as does Martha's. After two dismal prognoses from two separate doctors, I referred Martha to an oncologist who offered her hope by trying something new to overcome her rare cancer. She was doing well – a CAT scan showed her tumors were regressing, and she was feeling positive – but then she visited her naturopath who said, 'How are you confronting your mortality?', adding 'You *do* know that the drug you are on is the treatment of last resort?' This last statement was incorrect, but she did not know that, and the effect on her was devastating. Two months later she was dead.

6   There are alternative practitioners who claim that if you don't
    recover it is your fault because your belief was not strong
    enough. This can be crushing. The fact is that some people
    believe they will recover, yet they do not; equally, some people
    don't believe they will recover, and yet they do. Although it is
    highly important, belief is only an aid to, not a guarantee of,
    healing.

7   Some specialists do not treat the whole person, but the same
    could be said of some GPs and alternative practitioners. For
    example, the GP or alternative practitioner who gives you
    vitamin C injections and shark cartilage tablets in the belief
    that he can heal you is not treating you as a whole person, but
    attempting to treat your cancer symptoms.

The limits of any doctor

As long as people believe doctors can cure every disease, they are
bound to be disappointed. As long as they think that doctors are all-
knowing and all-powerful, they will tend to pick on them rather than
address the real problem. There are still some diseases for which
there are no cures. There are treatments that work better with some
people than others.

In my experience, both conventional and alternative practitioners
can – like cab drivers, teachers, politicians and electricians – be very
good, good, indifferent, bad and even downright stupid. If you can
accept this, you are more likely to be less disappointed in them if they
can't perform miracles. They, in turn, may feel more comfortable in
knowing that you understand this.

I have been fortunate in having an excellent cancer specialist who is
also humane, inspiring and comforting. Yet, I am aware that his power
to heal me is not limitless. My life has been saved on several occasions
as much by new medical technology as by a sharp-eyed doctor.

You need your doctor's skills and knowledge to keep your disease
under control; he needs your participation to achieve this. You are
unlikely to provide him with your willing co-operation unless you
get to know and respect him; he is unlikely to offer you the best treatment and care he can if he fails to get to know you. It is highly likely
that both of will feel let down if your expectations of each other fail
to match reality.

Building a therapeutic relationship

Building a therapeutic relationship with your doctor is essential to your eventual recovery, so it is vital you both recognise each other's strengths and limitations.

A therapeutic relationship is one in which your doctor accepts you as an *active*, not a *passive*, partner and, as I will explain in more detail in the following chapter, acknowledges that the role you adopt can improve your chances of survival. Your doctor can provide you with all the ammunition modern medicine has to offer, but it is up to you to decide whether you wish to fight or throw in the towel. You can bring out the best in your doctor if you ask the right questions and make it clear that you intend to take responsibility for yourself. It will make you feel more confident, and it will take the pressure off your doctor to 'perform'. Be prepared to take a risk. Be prepared to say 'No,' and 'I don't agree with you.'

A therapeutic partnership recognises that your body carries the miracle of healing from within as a natural function of the body's immune system. You and your doctor have shared responsibilities in this process. Defining your disease and the treatment needed to overcome it is your doctor's responsibility; regarding your disease as unacceptable and trying to get better as quickly as possible is yours.

For any given treatment, some people get better, others do not. There are many possible reasons for this. How far a disease has progressed before treatment can make a difference to the outcome, so an early diagnosis is better than a late one. Some cancers are slow-growing, others are aggressive; some treatments are effective, others are not. The skill of one doctor may be superior to that of another. The nursing care in one hospital may be more attentive and caring than in another. I believe, however, that your response to the challenge and the degree to which you retain control can help to tip the scales in your favour.

STARTING WITH REALISTIC EXPECTATIONS

A therapeutic relationship with your doctor will be difficult to achieve if your expectations of each other are unrealistic. For example, some people feel cheated if their doctors don't *do* something: hand them a prescription, send them for X-rays or blood tests. Yet if your doctor sends you for endless tests, a cycle of expectation and disappointment can be set in motion.

Television, the media and inadequate medical education are undoubtedly major causes of unrealised expectations. Many 'soapies' with a medical theme show someone with a serious disease rescued in the nick of time by an ever-present, all-knowing doctor. Ambulances arrive within moments of being called, heroic efforts at saving people are invariably successful, and patients seem stoic, cheerful and almost never in pain. It's a quite misleading picture. News reports, too, often raise unrealistic hopes with sensational accounts of discoveries in medical research, leading their readers and viewers to believe that the cure for a disease will be immediately available. For example, in 1997, as a result of media hype about a new cocktail of drugs to treat AIDS, many people believe the end of this dread disease is in sight. This novel treatment has succeeded in treating some cases, but it is so expensive that people with AIDS in those countries with the highest incidence of this disease cannot afford it.

False assumptions

If you leave every decision to your doctor he will, most certainly, make some or all of the following assumptions about you:

- You are a victim of circumstance.
- You have a negligible role to play in your recovery.
- You don't understand what is going on.
- You accept everything he tells you, and he knows everything about your particular condition.
- You accept your role as a passive spectator rather than as an active and interested participant, and so
- You don't wish to know anything about your condition or the treatments for it.
- You are prepared to be treated without any regard to your particular individual character, fears and expectations.
- You will blindly follow all his instructions, no matter how you feel about them.
- You believe that nothing will save you, so you will do as you're told as this is what your doctor and your family expect of you.

You may also make assumptions about your doctor that will do little to help you. For example, if your doctor acts decisively and appears to be in control, you may assume that he knows what he is doing. The opposite is often true: when people are unsure of what they are doing, they often take over in a manner designed to hide their uncertainty.

Your doctor should never assume that if you ask no questions you have no questions to ask. You may not have had the opportunity to ask, you may be afraid to ask in case you offend or upset him, and you may feel you don't know enough yet to ask the appropriate questions. If you've only just heard your diagnosis, you may be left momentarily speechless.

Some doctors assume that if you're quiet, then you're serene, complacent or, even worse, stupid. What many doctors fail to appreciate is that you may be scared to death; or you may be afraid to ask certain things for fear of offending him; or simply not sure how to frame the questions you need answers for. Some doctors assume you have some working knowledge of anatomy, so it's OK to use medical jargon; others that you know nothing so there's no point in even trying to explain it to you.

Your assumption may be that it is in your doctor's power to fix all your problems just as easily as a mechanic replaces a spark plug in your car. You may also assume that because your doctor doesn't spend much time with you, or keeps you waiting, he doesn't care about you, when it may be simply a matter of long waiting lists caused by funding shortfalls. (There is no doubt that economic policies in many countries have made it almost impossible for many doctors to practise good medicine – i.e. spend time with their patients; equally, unless doctors stand up for change, the situation will get worse.)

KEEPING CONTROL

The science of medicine is one you are unlikely to know much about but is the one in which your doctor has been well schooled. Not surprisingly, your doctor assumes that since only he knows how to decipher the tests you have undergone, only he knows what is best for you. The moment he makes this assumption – *and you allow him to act upon it without question* – control is taken away from you. The result is that you become dependent on him to make decisions on your behalf.

It **is** your doctor's responsibility to diagnose and manage your symptoms. It **is** your doctor who sends you to hospital and then sends you home. It **is** your doctor who orders up tests, prescribes medication and recommends surgery, chemotherapy or radiotherapy. Gradually, many doctors – even women doctors – can assume a paternalistic role. As you follow their blur of signals, you become spellbound and so lose even more control.

For most people, this is a terrifying ordeal. People who were in complete control of their lives suddenly find themselves dependent and fearful the moment they enter their doctor's consulting room. This is particularly true of the aged who are more marginalised than others by the paternalistic and patronising approach taken to them by their doctors.[2]

There are many people who hand control of their destiny to a doctor or alternative practitioner when they have been diagnosed with cancer, and are then angry and resentful when they are told what to do. They are often people accustomed to dealing with problems and making their own decisions, and they feel alienated when they are no longer asked for their opinion. If you find yourself being prodded and pricked by a retinue of experts with total power over your body, it is not unusual to feel indignant and helpless.

UNDERSTANDING EACH OTHER

Cancer is rarely treated in a one-off procedure. If you have a skin cancer removed, you may only need to see your doctor once a year for a check-up. In most cancer cases, though, treatment and check-ups require ongoing visits, so you will probably need to maintain contact with your doctor for weeks, months, even years. In the light of this, you both need to get along with each other in every way possible. Your doctor has to adopt a non-critical attitude and accept you for who you are.

Knowing more about your beliefs and values is essential learning on the part of your doctor. It will help him interpret your problems within *your* value system, not his, so that when it comes to discussing another course of treatment, he stands a better chance of meeting *your* needs and expectations. He is less likely to suggest treatment you don't wish to undergo, or force you to submit to extensive and invasive tests that distress you.

You expect your doctor to give you the best advice possible, and you will follow his advice *if* you respect his knowledge and his judgement. However, you are most unlikely to do so if he cannot put himself in your shoes, cannot appreciate how you feel about medical information and procedures, and especially if he conceals his lack of empathy behind a mask of arrogance. It is to your mutual benefit to build a therapeutic partnership that eliminates the imbalance between the doctor's paternalism and your dependence. No doctor should project his or her fear of failure or obsessive desire to fix the world onto you.

The fact is, doctors are not God, they are human. As humans, they have no real control over the final outcome. If they prescribe a course of treatment, they cannot control whether it will work or not. If it works, it isn't because they are God. If it doesn't work, it isn't because they are the Devil. Both you and your doctor need to recognise this fundamental fact.

Look for the Compassionate Doctor

The compassionate doctor is the one who can appreciate your suffering, and does whatever he can to relieve it. He understands that to show pity is an expression of fear, to show compassion is a sign of love; that to fulfil his calling as a doctor, he has to go beyond defined medical duties.

In her landmark book, *Living with Death and Dying*, Elisabeth Kübler-Ross points out that the most extreme anguish we can feel is to be forsaken and not to be heard; that we cope better if we are reassured that our doctors will not desert us.[3] The compassionate doctor will understand this and pay particular attention to your needs; he will never hide from his humanity by labelling you 'unhelpful' or 'un-co-operative', by calling your disease 'the worst of its kind I've ever seen' or blaming the system by saying something like, 'I'd like to help, but my hands are tied.' He will do what he can to allay your fears (and his) by accepting his role as your expert cancer guide, and he will help you work through and understand your illness. He will be aware how scary the buzz-words are that doctors use and how terrifying the paraphernalia and procedures of a hospital or treatment centre can be, so he will try to explain everything to you – and then check to make sure you understand.

Even if they go out of their way to choose the right words, doctors have to recognise that you may hear only what you want or don't want to hear. For example, your doctor may say, 'You need to undergo surgery,' but you hear, 'You don't need to undergo surgery.'

You need someone to listen to you, share your pain, your desolation, your despair, and your hopes. No one who truly appreciates your suffering will ever give you gratuitous advice, attempt to out-do you with their own personal experiences, make moral judgements about your behaviour, or try to be dogmatic. This can be extremely upsetting as it was for Richard, a man with lymphoma I once counselled who said to me, 'I feel as if I'm invisible to my doctor. He has no idea of how I feel. According to him most of my problems are in my head. All he does is tell me what he thinks.' Even now, as we approach the millennium, women tell me that male doctors show them little compassion, and regard their complaints as neurotic or 'all in the head'.

Most experienced doctors accept that modern science is limited in dealing with such a complex organism as a human being. The compassionate doctor will accept you as the person you are, not as someone defined by your illness – just as he is not (hopefully) defined by his profession but as the person he really is. Accepting that you have the right to be treated with consideration and with love, he will see you as a human being with a name – not as a case labelled 'the myeloid leukemia woman', or 'the motor neurone bloke'.

It is my hope that instead of doctors saying, 'We think we can cure frequently, relieve much of the time, and comfort when we get around to it,' they will say, 'We can cure frequently, relieve often, and comfort *always*.'

Look for the doctor with good bedside manners

The guiding spirit of modern medicine, Sir William Osler (1849–1919), once said, 'Medicine is learned by the bedside and not in the classroom.'

Good bedside manners start with the way your doctor talks to you, looks at you, and puts you at ease. Good bedside manners apply in your doctor's consulting room, a hospital ward, in a corridor, or on the phone.

The doctor with good bedside manners is the one who 'puts his backside on the bedside' so he is at eye level with you – and *keeps* looking at you while he talks. Eye-level contact shows he's interested in what you have to say. The doctor who can't look you in the eye has something to hide, be it his own fears, his uncertainty about how to communicate with you, his indifference towards you, or simply the fact that his thoughts are elsewhere.

The doctor with good bedside manners understands that maintaining his and your self-esteem are critical, so he will never attempt to dominate the conversation, either verbally or by body language – and he will be extremely careful to ensure he says nothing to cause you distress. He will always attempt to soothe your fears with a quiet word or the touch of a hand, but not treat you as if you were made of china – he'll have a sense of humour and be prepared to laugh and joke with you. If he's sensitive to your situation, he will know that being overly solicitous and unnaturally solemn can make him seem patronising.

The aged are particularly likely to be patronised. There is, perhaps, no clearer illustration of this than when a doctor says – perhaps with an arm around you – 'Hello Mrs Smith. How are *we* today?' You don't have to put up with this behaviour. Betty Thompson, a woman I once counselled, told me that whenever a doctor spoke to her in this fashion, she would reply, 'Don't you know how *you* are? I know how *I* am.'

Some doctors believe that if they become too friendly with their patients this will cloud their judgement when it comes to making clinical decisions. It may be difficult, under certain circumstances, for someone emotionally close to you to treat you, but if your doctor finds clinical detachment an emotional refuge in the face of human suffering, perhaps you ought to look for another doctor.

Look for the doctor who respects your individuality

The doctor who tells you there are no more options because he believes there are none denies you the opportunity to hold onto (or reclaim) your valuing of yourself as a person. Anyone who ignores your right to personal choice negates your individuality and perpetrates an act of emotional violence against you. If your doctor doesn't think you are worth the effort, how can you be expected to fight for your life?

The doctor who has your best interests at heart will always keep you informed, provide you with support, protect your dignity and independence, and help you explore options – for your cancer and yourself. People *feel* better when they are *treated* better. Your doctor needs to be as sensitive to your needs as those of your family. He should always try to give you a considered opinion about your condition and discuss this with you rather than attempt to persuade you to do what *he* wants.

It is your right to make whatever decision helps you to maintain your self-esteem. If your doctor acts with humility and tolerance of *your* definition of quality of life, he will recognise and accept this. It's hard to maintain your composure when everyone around you acts as if everything is OK and you believe you're dying; it's equally difficult to maintain your sense of purpose when everyone around you acts as if you're going to die and you believe you're not.

Look for the doctor with an open mind

When you are desperately ill and find yourself without hope, you are likely to seek out a sympathetic ear and a treatment you hope will cure you – even if you know, deep down, that the treatment is useless. From your point of view, 'Nothing ventured, nothing gained' can make the difference between living and dying.

The only way your doctor can prevent you from chasing rainbows is to allow you to explore other options – with his full co-operation and support; to act as an honest broker and steer you in the direction of the best possible help. Some doctors do keep an open mind to new possibilities and accept that patients can be legitimate sources of learning.

If your doctor understands your need to maintain your dignity and control over your life, he will accept that there are always options, including the option of doing nothing. The doctor I went to for a second opinion on my leukemia accepted that my determination to retain control over my life was as good an approach as any other. 'With your attitude,' he said, 'I have no doubt we'll toast your survival in a year's time.' His reassurance gave wings to my subdued optimism. So far, we've drunk fifteen toasts – and I hope will share many more.

The doctor with an open mind will also recognise that most people cannot face the thought of prolonged and severe pain. It is you, not your doctor, who has to choose whether you wish to endure pain – and for how long. As I will explain in more detail in Chapter 8, I believe that your doctor is obliged to offer you relief, however temporary, if it is available. Your ignorance should never be his excuse for not making the offer.

Try to read up as much as you can about your condition, the treatments available, and what other people have done when faced with a similar problem. If you don't understand some of the medical jargon, make a copy of the relevant article or paragraph and ask your doctor to explain it. If you've chosen the right doctor, he will never feel that you're challenging his knowledge or his trust. He will be impressed by your efforts, and will appreciate that you want to be actively involved in your recovery program. If your doctor refuses to explain an article you have found, for example, on a novel treatment for your cancer, or if he fobs you off with a comment like 'Oh, that's old hat!' or 'Why are you bothering with this?', find someone who will not only explain it to you, but will also tell you how it has been superseded (if it has), and by what. You have every right to be informed.

The doctor with an open mind will understand that cancer, heart disease and other life-threatening illnesses not only receive detailed media coverage but are often the subject of talk shows on radio and television. He will be aware that people are far more aware of the symptoms and variety of treatments available for most diseases. If he is attuned to this, he will keep himself informed of the latest advances and controversial issues, not only in his particular field, but in related disciplines.

The ultimate test of your doctor's openness is his preparedness to say, 'I don't know.' With all the promise of technology at their fingertips, we expect doctors to have all the answers; they, in turn, often believe they do. As you may already have discovered, there are exceptions. If your doctor admits he doesn't have a ready solution to your problem – and you see this as courage and not a weakness on his part – you have the opportunity for a candid relationship from which you both have much to gain and little to lose.

If your doctor is not up-to-date and open-minded, look for someone who is.

Look for the doctor who communicates

True communication starts with honesty – with the doctor telling you the whole truth and answering all your questions . If your doctor is aware of this, he will do his utmost to lead you to an accurate understanding of the significance of the diagnosis, and to an awareness of what he can or cannot do.

Only in this way will you both be clear where his responsibility ends and yours begins. It is not your doctor's function to decide what is an appropriate life or death for you. As such, he will never tell you he has 'bad news' for you. There are ways and ways of putting the facts to you. Your doctor needs to tell you the truth in a way that leads you, as gently as possible, to your own understanding of it. It's most unlikely that you will find the courage to struggle on if your condition is presented to you as terminal or as a crisis. If it's presented to you as a challenge, there's every chance it will bring out the fighting spirit in you.

The dangers of withholding information

The doctor who withholds vital information from you assumes a paternalistic role based on the following assumptions: that only he knows what is best for you, that you should not have any say in what you do or do not know, that you should not have any say in decisions about your diagnosis or treatment.[4]

Refusing to keep you informed is rendered a nonsense if the lump in your breast turns out to be cancerous and your doctor recommends surgery or radiotherapy. It's just as ridiculous if, despite your tiredness, loss of weight, and persistent cough, your doctor suggests a course of chemotherapy – and you know it's a standard treatment for cancer. If the information withheld is really basic – for example, if he does not tell you that your illness is, or is likely to be, cancer, or he does not tell you it is life-threatening – your doctor creates a whole set of problems.

1   You may not give him your full co-operation with treatment which could alleviate your symptoms.
2   You will be denied the choice of accepting or refusing treatment – and you certainly won't be able to choose between being an active participant or a passive spectator in your treatment program.

3   As a consequence of either the disease or the treatment you
     and everyone in your life – particularly young children – will
     struggle to adapt. You would have every right to feel angry if
     you suddenly find yourself asking for help to eat, to go to the
     bathroom or to get dressed – *and you don't know the real reason
     for your loss of control*. You would also have every right to feel
     angry if your pain and disability disrupted your sex life – *and
     you didn't know why*. Yet there are doctors who don't tell their
     patients that the lump in the breast in malignant, or that their
     tiredness suggests, for example, lung cancer.

4   If your cancer is life-threatening and you do not know it, you
     will be denied the opportunity to sort out your unfinished
     business and unresolved conflicts, whatever they are: patching
     up old squabbles, making a will and a 'living will', finding out
     about your social security entitlements, making sure your life
     insurance premiums are up to date, deciding whether to
     donate your organs or not, and saying farewell – by word or
     gift – to the people in your life who count.

5   You may find it extremely difficult to explain to your
     employer why you have to take so much time off, either for
     treatment or because you are too tired to work.

6   You may make risky decisions you'd not make if you knew –
     deciding to start a new business venture, say, or taking off on
     an overseas trip. Conversely, you may be deprived of the
     motivation to take risks that you *would* have wished to take –
     the trip you've been putting off for years, an examination of
     your rocky marriage, or whatever.

7   You may lose the opportunity to re-discover your long-lost
     faith or find a new one. Your doctor has no right to deny you
     the chance to delve into the mysteries of life and death.

8   You will be denied the opportunity to ask for help, love and
     support from your loved ones; they will be denied the
     opportunity to give them to you.

9   You will be prevented from searching out other opinions and
     from exploring other options, not necessarily for your
     treatment but for the way you want to live.

Cicely Saunders, the founder of the hospice movement in the United Kingdom, touched on the heart of the matter when she said, *'The truth from which the patient is protected is the truth from which he is being forced to live in isolation.'*

If you are deprived of full information, you are more likely to see your condition as a tragedy rather than an opportunity. If you see it as a tragedy, you are more likely to throw in the towel, leave all the decisions to your doctor or spouse (is that fair?) and give up. You may also conjure up images far worse than the reality, in which case there will be no way for you to relieve your fears.

Doctors' failure to tell the truth is one of the main reasons why people believe cancer is so deadly and why, if someone *does* recover, they say, 'Oh, he probably never had cancer in the first place/the diagnosis was probably wrong/they looked at someone else's X-rays!' If no one knew you had cancer and you suddenly died, the assumption would be that you were struck down before anything could be done for you: cancer is then seen as a swift and silent killer. If you were told you had cancer only when it was at an advanced stage and shortly afterwards you died, the assumption would be that the treatment was ineffective: cancer is then seen as an incurable disease. This kind of thinking ignores the high success rate of many cancer treatments and encourages a fatalistic attitude. It can also result in a delay in seeking help because of fear.

Studies confirm that most people want to be told the whole truth, whether their disease is considered curable or not,[5] although some feel they should be told only as much they need to know. In general, these studies reveal that people who are not told the full story feel isolated and become depressed, anxious and distrustful. One study found that doctors who tell their patients are the very ones who express the view that if they were the patient they would wish to be told.

In general, there are only two occasions when a doctor should consider withholding information from a patient:

1   if he is absolutely sure the patient's physical or mental health might be seriously harmed;
2   if a patient expressly asks him not to – in which case he is still obliged to provide basic information about the illness, and about proposed tests and treatments.[6]

Choosing the right words

Most people remember very little of what they've been told in dramatic circumstances, particularly when they have been told they have a life-threatening illness. Your doctor has to choose his words carefully, speak to you in language you understand, and check with you constantly to make sure you grasp what he has told you.

The art of skilful communication is vital to good medicine at all times. This is especially important when your doctor discusses your treatment program with you. He owes it to you to make sure you not only understand what he has said — but that you understand the implications.

Look for the doctor who listens

Long before a doctor can assess whether you want to hear the truth or whether you are strong enough to handle it, he has to find out more about you. To do so, he must strive to be an empathic listener. If he's smart, he'll button his lip and encourage you to talk. How else can he know what you really feel? Just listening to your questions can make a world of difference — even if he doesn't have the answers.

The doctor who really listens, listens with both ears: one attuned to what you say and the other to what you don't say — even your silences can speak volumes about the way you feel. The doctor who listens understands that you need time — and he gives you time — to absorb and respond to what he discusses with you. A single session is usually too short to allow adequate discussion of treatment and available options.

The opportunity to establish good communications is lost when you are discouraged from asking questions and when you feel rushed. You are bound to feel less important if your doctor interrupts you while you are talking or asking questions. No one can talk and listen at the same time.

Look for the doctor with humility

If he has acquired some wisdom, your doctor will recognise that
☞ he has limitations as well as strengths;
☞ he has the potential for disease within himself and is also mortal;

- ☞ there is much he does not know;
- ☞ he can only diagnose and manage your symptoms, knows healing is one of life's miracles; and
- ☞ that any compulsion he feels to be in control is a mask behind which to hide his own fears.

The right doctor

So who is the right doctor? Here's how I'd summarise it.

- ☞ He's the one who is prepared to listen to you, share what he knows with you, regards *care* and *cure* in the same light, and who will always continue to comfort you when he finds he cannot relieve your symptoms.
- ☞ He's the one who knows that the more time he spends with you and the closer he gets to you, the better his chance of making the right diagnosis and suggesting the most appropriate course of treatment for you.
- ☞ He's the one who treats you as a whole person and is as concerned about your dignity as your health. He's the one who does not patronise you and never speaks to you in that tone of voice that keeps you at arm's length.
- ☞ He's the one who recognises you are an individual with feelings and says, 'Hello, Mrs Jones. How are *you* today?' – and says it with feeling.
- ☞ He's the one who believes in honesty, and when he can't find the right words, admits he doesn't know what to say.
- ☞ He's the one who explains things clearly, projects confidence in his ability and matches your needs.

Choose someone who cares, someone you like, someone you can trust, someone who knows what they're doing – and why.

Part Two

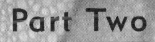

the road to

recovery

five

how to be a survivor

Seeing yourself as a survivor

In any life-threatening situation, most people adopt one of two basic responses. One is to say, 'That's it! I've had it.' The other is to say, 'How do I get out of here?' The second response is the response of a survivor; it will lead you to take stock of your situation and then decide on the best course of action.

To commute what you believe could be a sentence of death into a sentence of life, you have to see yourself as a survivor; you have to picture yourself getting past this point of danger. But you can't make this mental shift until you understand more about yourself, your disease and your treatment options.

To begin with, you need information; you have to find out what is the best treatment for your condition – with due regard to side effects, length of treatment, cost of treatment, long-term prospects and, most importantly, quality of life.

If you feel you are not equipped to meet the challenge of such inquiry, consider this: most of us use only a fraction of our potential until we have to, when self-preservation forces us to take action. It is only when we are confronted by the prospect of dying that we attempt to redefine ourselves and give meaning to our lives. The most valuable insights come as a result of the shock of a dramatic event – especially a cancer diagnosis, when we discover, to our amazement, that it is not so much who we are that matters, but rather *what we are able to be.*

If we acknowledge that we all have untapped potential, we can rise to the challenge of a cancer diagnosis. One of the most valuable survival lessons I learned is that you can't always change the situation in which you find yourself, *but you can change your response to it.* You can choose to be a survivor.

What does survival mean to you?

When you ask people with cancer what the word 'survive' means to them, you'll get many different answers.

'Surviving past the treatment.'

'Seeing my daughter graduate from high school.'

'Making it until tomorrow.'

'Living for a long time to come.'

'Being out of pain.'

'Getting through the treatment.'

'Watching my children growing up.'

In general, people diagnosed with cancer have difficulty imagining a time when they will be healthy again, and doing what they love most. Those who survive are almost always those who can conjure up a picture of ongoing living. To help you believe in a future in which you can see yourself very much alive, you need to maintain hope, remain determined to retain your individuality and fulfil your dreams, and discover what healing means (see Chapter 6). In the face of a shortened life span, you are more likely to become aware of what really matters, make every effort to restore the balance in your life, take responsibility for getting well again.

Choice and meaning

There's no more radical catalyst than a cancer diagnosis to make you aware of the gift of choice. Choosing gives you a sense of purpose and renewed strength. However, you can't make choices unless you understand what is happening to you, and to be informed, you need to ask questions – no matter how silly you may think they are – and you need to challenge your doctors to find the answers.

In the process of gathering information, survivors look around for help. Reaching out for help is natural, but if, in the process, you permit others to make decisions for you, you become dependent on them: you become a patient. Unfortunately, many of those around you – your spouse, your doctor, your family – equate taking care with taking charge. You need to be in charge, not them.

There is rarely an excuse for saying, 'But it's all too hard to understand!' As I will explain in Chapter 9, your doctor has a legal and moral obligation to answer all your questions in a way you do understand. If he or she won't, find someone who will.

I have listed some basic questions in Chapter 2, and more in Chapter 6. If you follow up by researching your disease, you will know what further questions to ask. I also have included a Resource Guide at the back of the book to help guide you through the maze. Remember, too, that there are medical libraries attached to all teaching hospitals.

Once you understand the choices available to you, you can not only take charge of your treatment and thereby enhance your survival prospects, you can also decide what things have most meaning for you. When your life is on the line, you appreciate that most of the things you once considered important are really quite irrelevant; many of the things to which you attached little or no importance now occupy much of your attention. A life-shortening diagnosis compels you to give a new meaning to your life – for however long you live – and gives you the opportunity to realise your dreams.

The dangers of not taking the initiative

The thought of researching treatments and being assertive with your doctor may seem too much; your response may be 'I have cancer, and as if that weren't enough, you want me to take on more!'

The obvious way to get unstuck from your feeling of helplessness is to focus on what *you* want – not what your doctor, your family or your friends want. It is a folly to act out of ignorance. Your doctor may believe she knows all about your condition and has all the answers. If so, her views about treatment (or no treatment) will be based on *her* value system and what *she* deems appropriate.

From your doctor's point of view, your tacit agreement sends a signal to her that you accept this state of affairs and wish to play no part in decision-making. If you do feel like this, your opportunity to make your own meaning of your condition will be slim. On the other hand, if you choose to become an active director in your own drama, rather than a passive spectator, you will greatly increase your chances of survival. To want to know is to want to live; to leave everything to your doctor and ask no questions is to deny your potential and your ability to rise to the challenge. This inactivity could prevent you from gaining the kind of information essential to your prospects of survival, and take away the opportunity to make your own meaning out of your condition.

Everyone is different

Just as no two people are alike, no two cancers are alike. Your breast or colon cancer is not the same as someone else's. A doctor may tell you she has treated cases like yours, but the important difference lies in the word *like*. Like means similar – *not the same*. If pressed to explain this, doctors will admit that no two people present their cancers in the same way, and no two people respond to treatment in the same way.

Some people are allergic to penicillin, most are not; some people react badly to chemotherapy, many more do not. Some people respond to certain treatments which have no effect on others. To maximise your chances of recovery, you and your doctor have to be sure the treatment you are about to receive is the treatment you want to receive – because it is the most appropriate for *you*.

How your attitude can influence your prospects of survival

Most Western-educated doctors accept that the way to treat disease is through the mechanical and scientific model they have been taught. In this view, there is little or nothing you can do to influence the course of your disease.

Your own experience and intuition will tell you this is not true. Your emotional states *can* trigger physical reactions. When you're angry, your face turns red. When you're nervous, your hands sweat, your tummy gets upset. When you're embarrassed, your cheeks flush. When you're excited, your heart beats faster. When you're confused or anxious, you feel dizzy. If you acknowledge even a few of these mind-body connections, you'll realise your attitude does have a role to play in your recovery. Indeed, science itself is now researching the influence of psychological and social events on illness and recovery. Modern research on the mind-body connection has benefited from both increasing knowledge of how the immune system works and the ability to measure immune function.[1] I explain this in more detail further on.

Recognising that the solution to every problem is contained within the problem itself will help you take charge. The confidence that it will generate will give you what many people with cancer call 'cancer freedom' – that state of liberation where you can focus on only what really matters in life.

Cancer is a condition where the orderly pattern of cell reproduction gets out of control and invades its host body. Where once there was order, there is now dis-order; where once there was natural harmony, there is now anarchy.

The way to respond to the problem is to restore order. Cancer is not an invasion by an alien enemy; it is a sign of internal unrest. If you recognise this fact, you will appreciate that your role is significant in the treatment provided by your doctor – which is aimed at restoring order.

Spontaneous remissions and miracles do occur, and doctors know this, even when they do not acknowledge this openly. They also know that the attitude people bring into their treatment often makes a difference to the outcome. Your psychological response is a key aspect of survival.

The importance of maintaining hope

If you are afraid or in pain, your anguish becomes immediately bearable the moment you believe the end is in sight, the situation reversible, rescue possible.

Hope blows away despair. Hope can keep you going in the face of the most impossible odds. Your hope may assume any of several different shapes: that there are still options to explore, that your cancer is still treatable; that you will still be able to do the things you enjoy doing, and will not be isolated from those you love. Yet, what are doctors to do when science and experience tells them the situation is grim?

I believe it is possible to negotiate 'the facts' and provide comfort without creating unrealistic expectations. My own story is a case in point. The doctor who told me that there was no cure for my disease dropped me into a pit, but as soon as he told me that removing my spleen would 'buy me a little time', he gave me a glimmer of hope – enough to keep me going – even though he didn't believe I could be cured. As Dr William Osler, the father of modern medicine, said, 'It is not for you to don the black cap and, by assuming judicial function, take hope away from any patient.'

Only you can define the meaning of the word 'hope' for yourself. Different people hope for different things. You may want relief from pain, someone else a long and happy life; you may hope for a better relationship with your spouse, someone else may hope to die with dignity.

You are not a statistic

Your doctor condemns you to death when she tells you how long she thinks you have to live. If you believe there is no way out, no rescue, and if you find the thought of prolonged and unending suffering unendurable, the only escape from the situation becomes death itself. I believe this helps to explain why some patients die before their time. Those who feel helpless and consider their condition hopeless give up their resistance to dying while others in the same situation keep up hope and the will to live.

When your doctor attempts to formulate an outline of the course she believes your disease will take, she does so in order to plan a treatment program for you. If, on the other hand, she relies on statistics to predict how long you have to live, she ignores some fundamental issues.

Statistics are patterns of numbers, they are about groups of people, not individuals. As Professor Hinton points out in his book *Dying*, one of the factors influencing the survival of American prisoners of war by the Japanese was their decision to 'retain a sense of some individuality'.[2] You may present all the classical symptoms of a disease to your doctor, but your age, your sex, your lifestyle, your physical fitness, the stage of your disease and the extent of its spread (if any), the different approaches towards treatment adopted by different doctors, plus the type and quality of the hospital you're in, means the outcome for you will be different from the outcome for someone else with the same disease. If you add to all these factors your support system, attitude, optimism and individual will to live, any forecast a doctor makes is likely to be wrong.

In the light of spontaneous remissions where people recover for no apparent reason (although there are usually many reasons) and of amazing new discoveries in medicine – to say nothing of that indefinable will to live that some people exhibit more strongly than others – why do some doctors dare to put a time limit on their patients' lives? The reason, I believe, is that science demands precision, people expect their doctors to know the answer to everything, and cancer is still viewed by most people, including doctors, as a generally fatal disease.

In reality, many people have been cured of every type of cancer. Every type of cancer can be treated. There are innumerable, well-documented cases of people who have defied the odds and hung on to life well past the moment of their expected demise.

The following points are worth noting:

1   To statisticians, it makes little difference to their graphs whether an individual dies in one given year or another; to you it may make all the difference in the world – especially if treatment results in the bonus of years of productive, pain-free and enjoyable life.

2   Only you can choose whether you are prepared to be treated as a statistic or a person. If, for example, the choice of treatment for you consists of giving you five different injections that cause nausea, low blood counts, hair loss and other side effects, or giving you tablets with fewer side effects – but the former treatment is preferred because *according to statistical evidence* it will provide you with another three months of life, you have to ask yourself what trade-off you are prepared to make between time gained and side effects.

3   The course of some diseases – such as rabies and measles – can be predicted with accuracy. Bacterial infections of the heart and tuberculous meningitis progress rapidly and are generally fatal. On the basis of this knowledge, death or recovery from these conditions usually occur within a reasonably predictable

period. The course of diseases such as coronary heart disease, rheumatoid arthritis and cancer can only be generally outlined. Some people may only survive for one or two years, others for fifteen or more. This is an important point: there are so many variables in the case of cancer and diseases of the heart, kidney and brain due to arteriosclerosis that they cannot be listed in any textbook.

The implication of this is that unless she has encountered *every* form and *every* variable of these diseases (an impossible task), no doctor can ever be 100 per cent certain what the outcome will be unless death is hours away.

4   When your doctor tells you that you have, for example, Stage III or Stage IV Hodgkin's disease, she is measuring your disease mechanically. She cannot measure how you feel, so she has to assess the disease as something separate from you. The purpose of staging is to work out how to manage your disease – it is **not** to determine how long you have to live.[3] Dealing in hard facts does not take into account your intense passion to survive; dealing in numbers does not recognise the immeasurable value of hope. Your doctor has to estimate how long she needs to treat you – **not** how long she thinks you have to live. No doctor should ever take away your hope and sense of purpose by telling you how long you have to live. The doctor who puts a time limit on your life is being unnecessarily cruel – and actually reduces your chance of survival![4]

We all want to live long and disease-free lives. The ideal and the norm are two separate notions: in an ideal world, no one gets ill; in the real world perfect, disease-free health is granted to very few. There are some diseases, mainly viral, for which there are no known cures, no effective treatments. However, if you ignore the facts and figures, follow your heart instead of a strict diet, you may become so preoccupied with living the life you want to live, that you survive beyond your wildest expectations, find you can exert more control over your life than you thought possible, and get more out of it than if your days were numberless.

We all have the capacity and the creativity to give meaning to our lives. At no time do we have more freedom to do so than when we have been told we have a life-threatening disease: this is a time when *anything* is possible.

This is, indeed, what many people discover in the days after their diagnosis, when they realise they are still alive, that the shock of the news hasn't killed them, that they still have a future, though of possibly shorter duration. This is, initially, a dilemma, when you ask, 'What do I do now?' The way through the fog of panic is to stop, consider your options and choose that course of action with which you feel most comfortable.

Lessons to be learned from stories of survival

You can turn yourself from a victim of passive suffering into an active observer of your own condition and so regain some control of your life if, instead of seeing yourself overpowered by events, you detach yourself mentally from them and make them the object of your intellectual curiosity. As Cohen & Taylor point out in their book, *Psychological Survival,*[5] understanding what is happening to you is a fundamental rule for survival in all situations produced by events such as imprisonment, internment, tornadoes, volcanoes, hurricanes and shipwrecks. As long as you are alive you can influence what happens to you, and try to make whatever choices you need to enhance your chances of survival. One story particularly illustrates this point.

In 1982, a sailor's boat struck an unknown object, perhaps a whale, as he sailed from the Canary Islands to the West Indies. His boat capsized and sank in less than a minute. He managed to inflate his life raft and recover a few clothes and a ditch-kit. Even though he was a skilled sailor, nothing in his previous experience had prepared him for this event. After the initial shock of the accident wore off, one part of his mind screamed out, 'I'm going to die!' Another part screamed out, 'Shut up! Do this! Do that!'

And that's exactly what he did. Living from moment to moment he set himself little tasks, dividing each day into a manageable survival routine made up of exercise, navigation, writing up his log, reflecting on his life – and fishing. He was inspired to battle on by the thought that others had survived even tougher situations. His goal was to stay alive. Keeping a log ensured that he would have a record on which to base the story of his miraculous recovery should he survive the ordeal.[6] Stranded 1000 km from the nearest land, he lived on rainwater and the fish he caught with a makeshift speargun. After fighting off sharks and watching nine ships pass him by, he was finally rescued – 76 days later.

The survival value of setting yourself a goal is reinforced by the story of concentration-camp survivor and psychiatrist, Viktor Frankl. To get himself through each day in the face of the horrors around him, he imagined himself standing before a large audience and lecturing them on what he was experiencing at that precise moment. In this unique way, he came to understand what he was going through and was able to diarise his internment in his mind. Frankl survived and succeeded in realising his goal.[7] In my own case, I noted my thoughts and feelings daily in my diary as I was dying. Weary and ill as I was, I persisted in the belief that if I survived I would use my notes to write a book. My first book, *Time of My Life*, was published eight years later.

I and many others see a similarity between people facing a diagnosis of cancer and those who were sent to concentration camps during World War II. Psychiatrists, sociologists and concentration-camp survivors (Bettelheim, Frankl, Bluhm, Hinton, Cohen and Taylor, for example) concur that those who were selected for slave labour, weak and fearful as they were, saw in this short reprieve the hope that they might survive for even a few more hours or days; that somehow, events might change course in that time.[8] Others saw death as the only way out of something far worse to come, and threw themselves against electric fences.

Even a few weeks can be enough to come to an understanding and an acceptance, however uneasily and unhappily, that although we have to face death eventually, there is always the hope and the possibility that we may live a little longer. Survivors of the camps tell how they kept their hopes alive by imagining a goal, a life after their release (Bettelheim, Frankl). They dreamed of the things they would do when they were reunited with their parents or their children; they planned projects – one (Bettelheim) even interviewed his fellow inmates with a view to publishing his findings when he was eventually liberated. The internal search to make sense of what was happening was what gave them a reason to continue. Frankl makes the point that they gained strength from knowing that their hopes and dreams could not be taken away from them and so, with these intact, they did not break down.

A story closer to home reflects a similar attitude. An aunt of mine was diagnosed with lung cancer when she was 35 and her son five. Following surgery to remove one of her lungs, her doctor told her that he wasn't sure whether he had 'caught it in time', and that her condition was 'terminal'.

'I think you should make arrangements for your son's future,' he said.

'And who do you think is going to bring him up?' she asked.

'You have lots of brothers and sisters,' he replied.

'That may be so,' she said, 'but given what I've seen of the way they're bringing up their children, I wouldn't let any one of them near my son!' She added, 'I'll bring him up myself.'

She died 35 years later, one month after her son's first child was born. She also outlived the doctor who made the prediction!

Some people think it's too late to do anything, that they don't have the resources, or that they have nothing to look forward to; others feel that prolonging their lives will place emotional and financial burdens on their families – they feel guilty that those they used to care for may now have to care for them. As Louis Pasteur once noted, 'Fortune favours the prepared mind.' If you can look at your possibilities rather than your limitations, you will soon realise there are always things you can do to keep your hopes and dreams alive. As my aunt found out, you can have cancer and still live a long and fruitful life. It is possible to have a life-threatening disease and still feel healthy.

Every case of survival reveals the importance of strengthening your resolve rather than your muscles. There is a vast body of evidence to substantiate the fact that when people are diagnosed with cancer, forced into a concentration camp or sentenced to prison for life, they can draw inspiration from the knowledge that others have survived similar ordeals, stimulate their will to live by setting goals, and sustain themselves with the strength they gain from making meaning out of life instead of seeing life as having lost its meaning.

You have no idea how you well you can respond until you meet a life-threatening situation.

Survival and belief

Some people are comforted and sustained through their ordeals by a belief, often religious, that they will be protected or saved from harm. The diagnosis of a life-threatening disease often calls these beliefs into question; they feel that they are being punished for failing to be true to their faith, for having no faith at all, or for committing some misdemeanour or other.

Most cancer survivors, however, say that cancer has taught them something new about themselves, compelled them to reassess their priorities, revalue themselves, and review their relationships with family, friends, nature and God (however defined). They regard every day as a bonus, try to make the most out of each moment and live in the present – with one eye to a future near enough to set realistic goals. Many have found a peace of mind that had eluded them before. Not surprisingly, these cancer survivors say, 'Cancer was the best thing that happened to me.'

Being positive

It is essential to your survival to understand what is happening to you, but you have to translate what you discover into some form of positive action that enhances your capacity for survival. This has to come from within you. Consider the sayings, 'Take things one day at a time' and 'I must be positive.' Affirmations such as these can only be meaningful if they are expressions of a belief system you understand and actively embrace – as part of your own personality and your convictions. Other people telling you to 'think positively' can actually make you feel even more helpless and distressed.

It is normal after a cancer diagnosis to undergo a confusion of feelings, almost all of which contain an element of despair. It is essential that you honour these feelings so the process of psychological adjustment can occur. It is cruel of others to blame you for not being positive if, despite your best efforts and those of your doctor, your disease progresses. You are bound to feel the situation is hopeless and give up.

What do people mean when they say, 'You have to be positive'? Do they mean you should concentrate on only the good aspects of your life? Focus on a positive outcome? Not talk about death in their presence? Not give up?

I would define 'being positive' not as a single idea but as a belief system based on the following key elements.

1 DENIAL – that you will die when doctors or statistics say you will.

2 HOPE – that your treatment works, that a new treatment is found, that you will live to fight another day. Hope is actively imagining a future based on a realistic assessment of the present. Hope is thinking about life, rather than death.

3 OPTIMISM – a recognition that for every down there is an up, that you are not to blame for your disease, that even if your cancer is terminal, you are not. Hope and optimism can keep you going in the face of the most daunting odds, give you time to respond to treatment, give your body time to heal.

4 LOVE – an acceptance of who you are, plus an ability to be open to the love expressed to you by your family and friends, and to embrace the love of the spirit within you.

5 COMMITMENT TO ACTION – a determination to act rather than react. You have to take the first step – every pilgrimage demands it. Only you can decide if the end is worth the effort. If you do, you have to exhaust every option open to you. The greatest risk of all is to take no risk at all.

6 STILLNESS – to help you find the path to another knowing. By and large, most people have lost the ability to sit quietly alone, be with themselves. With so many distractions, we no longer hear the voice of our intuition or give our non-verbal talents time to engage.

7 HUMOUR – to help you maintain a sense of balance. Laughter is good medicine.

8 UNDERSTANDING that knowledge leads to choices, choices lead to freedom. Understanding is a prelude to action. You can't fight your disease simply by wishing it away or relying solely on your doctors. You need to learn as much about yourself and your disease as possible, decide what you want to do, go for it.

9 BELIEF – that you *will* get better, you *will* live for another day, you *will* win.

10   TRUST – that you are not alone, that your doctor will do her
      best to help you, and that nature always tries to maintain
      harmony by healing.

Normal dependence vs loss of autonomy

The *Oxford English Dictionary* defines independence as 'not being
subject to the authority of another'. Prior to your diagnosis, there
were times when you turned to your spouse, parents, children or
friends for support. Dependence of this sort is normal; there is no reason to change things now that you have been diagnosed with cancer.

There is, however, a difference between normal dependence and
surrendering your autonomy and control of your life. There is a difference between your letting your spouse speak out on your behalf
and him or her doing so without your consent. Your doctor should
never take the responsibility of making decisions for you unless you
have agreed to this beforehand.

There are some occasions, an emergency perhaps, when you may
have no choice; it's another thing to rely on others when you are capable of doing things yourself. When doctors and nurses take over the
decision-making process from you by telling you what to do, what to
wear and which way to turn, you have been transformed from a
human being into a part on an assembly line.

Many caregivers – including spouses, doctors and nurses – find
themselves empowered when they find you totally dependent on
them. If your helplessness gives them power over you, gives them a
new-found mission in life, makes them feel important, they may
attempt to prevent you from regaining your independence. There's a
fine line between having a supportive circle of family, friends and
doctors and being completely under their control. This may appear
quite normal to you, especially if you are a person who has spent your
life allowing other people to make decisions for you. If the passive,
supporting role was your style before, now is your chance to exercise
your choices – and to be heard.

Caregivers who say, 'I can't stand by and do nothing' need to
appreciate that by taking over they make it hard for you to maintain
some degree of independence, and you could end up paying for
it with your life. Similarly, people who use illness as their only

guarantee of gaining – and holding – attention have little reason to want to get better and so stand little chance of surviving.

The value of being independent of spirit

What does independence of spirit mean in terms of survival? Does it make any difference if you choose to let everyone else take care of you or decide to take care of yourself?

You may be compelled to depend on others for your physical well-being, but this does not mean you have to surrender control of your thoughts, feelings, dreams, and expectations.

Making your own decisions keeps you in control so that whatever decision you make is based on what *your* own intellect and *your* own intuition have combined to tell you. No matter how trivial the decisions you make may appear to you or to others – even choosing what you want to eat or how you want to dress – it can help you regain your sense of independence.

If you know deep down inside that there is something you can do for yourself but prefer not to, look at your possible motives:

☞ Are you surrendering your autonomy in order to gain attention you believe you would not receive under normal circumstances?

☞ Are you passing responsibility onto someone else in order to punish them for some wrong – real or imagined – they have inflicted upon you?

☞ Are you doing nothing because you feel that since you're paying someone else they should do the work?

There is ample evidence that choosing to be independent reflects a positive choice, with positive results. A well-known study at King's College Hospital, London, was conducted on a number of women who had undergone mastectomies and were considered likely to have a recurrence of their disease. According to the answers gathered by the interviewing psychiatrist, they were graded as having a powerful, little or no fighting spirit. More than ten years later, those who were categorised with a strong fighting spirit proved to have a greater chance of survival and being free of their disease than those who had little or no fighting spirit.[9] Other patient studies found that women who were passive, stoic and helpless did not do as well as those who were stubborn and took an interest in their recovery.[10]

In my own case, when I realised no one was coming to my rescue, I refused to surrender and actively searched for a solution to my problem. Although none of the alternative therapies I tried made any difference to my physical condition, my stubbornness kept me going long enough for a new treatment to become available. To do so, I had to make decisions, not wait for someone else to make them. Despite my confidence being challenged at every turn, I firmly believed I still had a life to live.

Those who believe they are worth saving are more likely to remain survivors. Those who feel they are worthless and are accustomed to getting other people to do things for them are unlikely to find the courage to endure the struggle. I have counselled many patients who have taken this view, few as extreme as that adopted by Robin.

The warning sign was simple and sudden: a pain in the chest. At first Robin's doctor thought he might have cracked a rib laughing with me a few days earlier. Two days later, the pain unrelieved by analgesics, he went for X-rays and was diagnosed with a type of cancer that usually responds well to two or more rounds of chemotherapy.

The first round left him weak, depressed, bald. His doctor pointed out the advantage of starting a second round within a few days, but Robin convinced himself it would be a waste of time, went home, surrounded himself with family and friends, and prepared to die. His condition deteriorated so rapidly and his discomfort became so intense that he agreed to recommence treatment. His doctor told me he was puzzled at Robin's delay, and could not understand why he chose not to fight. Robin later told me that, despite his career success, he felt he wasn't worth saving, and feared disgrace when people realised his recent work was not up to his previous high standards.

I believe we are responsible for our attitude and our behaviour at all times. Responsibility has nothing to do with blame or guilt, rather with accepting that you are the author of your choices. By willing yourself to act, you free yourself to discover and acknowledge the power you have within you, start believing in yourself again, realise you are worth saving. Exercising your freedom of choice is likely to help you create new opportunities for yourself. If you were afraid to strike out in the past because you were fearful of being seen as a failure – in your own eyes and those of others – now is your chance to trust your instinct, assert your independence, create a climate of survival, respond to that inner call to life.

We never know how much we can do until we have to. A hero and a coward are both afraid. The difference between them is that the hero overcomes his fears, the coward is overwhelmed by them. The opposite of fear is not fearlessness, but courage.

six

weighing up alternatives

'Medicine can fend off death,
but in so doing it often prolongs the agony.'

Dr Robert Morrison[1]

Decision time

Your doctor has to consider a number of key issues before he can suggest a treatment program to you: your particular type of cancer, its size, whether it has metastasised (spread), its predicted response to various treatments, the hospital with the best nursing and equipment, and of course, the intended goal: to cure your disease or ease your symptoms, or both. He also has to take into account your age, your overall state of health, your attitude, and the cost if you are a fee-paying patient.

You, too, have to consider many factors – and become informed about the issues. Like many people, you may have preconceived notions about chemotherapy or radiotherapy but not much knowledge. You may believe that cancer is always fatal, that radiotherapy and chemotherapy are useless and always have side effects, usually bad. You may also have to bear with the prejudices and fears of family and friends, especially if they are concerned about your time away from work and urge you to start treatment immediately without considering its long-term effects.

Before you can agree to your doctor's recommendations, you have to consider a number of issues. The operative word is 'agree' because, as you will discover in this chapter and the next, you may have many more choices – and possibly better prospects – than you thought. You need time to think – with clarity and without background clatter – before you consent to treatment. You also need information: the more you know, the easier it will be to make an informed decision. For instance, a general rule doctors follow is: 'The better the chance of a cure or prolonging life, the more intense the treatment.' Moreover, some tests take longer than others to analyse, so your doctor may apply a second therapy – such as a round of antibiotics or steroids – in addition to the main treatment while he prepares a full treatment program for you. He might do this, for example, to prevent the possibility of a serious infection that could affect the outcome of your primary treatment.

Questions to ask your doctor about treatment

Many people dwell on the nastier side effects of medical treatment without realising that *the side effects of having no treatment are invariably worse*. It is important you remind yourself of this, or you could miss out on agreeing to a treatment that would prolong your life.

The questions below are designed to reveal your doctor's intentions and provide you with enough information to make an informed decision.

- What is the purpose of the treatment: rid me of my cancer (cure) or control the symptoms (palliate)?
- What are the benefits/disadvantages of your suggested treatment over any other?
- What will it cost?
- How long will the treatment take? How long will the sessions be, and over what period will they take place?
- What are the names of the drugs you recommend?
- Will the treatment have to be repeated at a later stage?
- What happens if I miss a treatment?
- If I have no side effects, will this mean the treatment did not work?
- What other medications or treatments will I have to take or receive?
- Will I need a blood test or any other tests before you start treatment?
- Will I have to have these tests afterwards as well – and when?
- Are there side effects of these tests? What are they likely to be – and how can you control them?
- Are there any foods I will have to avoid?

- ☞ Will I be allowed to drink any alcohol? What can I drink?
- ☞ Will I be able to conceive and have children?
- ☞ Will I retain the right to cancel out at any time?
- ☞ Is the treatment part of a trial? If so, what is the standard treatment and how effective is it? And why are you recommending that I try the new one?
- ☞ Is the treatment part of a trial – or is there a current trial for which I am eligible?
- ☞ What will happen if I don't have any treatment?
- ☞ What other options are there?

Remember you should always have the right to withdraw from treatment without being told 'You're being foolish', 'It's not the done thing', 'I wouldn't do that if I were you.' After all, the person about to undergo treatment is you, not your family, not your doctor. With regard to the last question your doctor should know what other treatments are available. If he can't suggest anything, ask him to refer you to another cancer specialist or a cancer centre where clinical trials may be under way. These centres are located in major hospitals.

Questions to ask yourself before deciding on treatment

DO I WANT TO BE TREATED TO DEATH?

Are you prepared to undergo, for example, a number of operations that may have no, or little, effect on your recovery? Are you prepared to face any number of procedures that are designed to manage your symptoms but will have no long-term effect on your condition?

In my own case, the doctor who eventually diagnosed my cancer wanted to remove my spleen. I declined his offer when I realised that surgery was intended only to prevent potential symptoms, but was not a cure. That was a long time ago – and I still have my spleen.

DO I WANT TO LIVE AT ANY COST – EVEN IF THERE IS NO QUALITY TO MY LIFE?

There may be a number of procedures that would enable you to gain a few extra months, an extra year, possibly more; but they may cause very unpleasant side effects.

Are you prepared to undergo these treatments, in the hope that they will prolong your life, even if they destroy the quality of that life? Only you can make this decision.

WHAT SUPPORT CAN I EXPECT IF I DO WHAT I WANT TO DO?

Are you following your doctor's advice because you made up your own mind to do so, or because of pressure by your family? Will there be someone to care for you if you choose to undergo prolonged and painful treatment? Are you likely to encounter hostility or rejection from your spouse, parents, family or friends if you choose to forgo all treatment because you don't want to suffer any side effects or feel that any treatment will only prolong your misery?

Family members often need reminding that *you* are the patient, *your* choice is the one that matters. If you choose to take responsibility for your decisions (and I believe you should) you will gain strength if your family and friends support your decisions, not criticise them.

WHAT IS THE SUCCESS RATE OF THE TREATMENT MY DOCTOR HAS SUGGESTED?

Many people go along with their doctor's decision without satisfying themselves as to the possible outcome of that decision. You owe it to yourself to ask as many questions as possible. People are often either too shy or too embarrassed to ask their doctors if they've treated cases like theirs before – and with what success. Unquestioning trust can often have painful consequences.

DO I WANT TO EXPLORE OPTIONS AND THEN DECIDE?

A second, third or even fourth opinion can give you the opportunity to examine several options and choose the way you want to live.

Some people say how painful they find it to watch the 'hopeless struggle'[2] of patients who refuse certain treatments or seek help from a whole array of 'alternative' practitioners when they feel that their doctors are not curing them. It may indeed be painful to watch, but what these people fail to recognise is that the search is an expression of the will to live and the right to decide for oneself.

It is your right to seek out a second or even a third opinion if your doctor isn't making any headway. Why shouldn't you abhor drugs that dull your senses? Why shouldn't you refuse palliative treatment if it won't cure or even prolong your life – especially if this entails the pain of surgery?

Your intuition may tell you there is little your doctor can do to alleviate your pain or treat your condition. If a further opinion confirms this, and you choose to refuse all treatment – and this is a legitimate choice – your doctor and family have to respect your decision. Maintaining your dignity and determination to retain control over your life takes precedence over all other considerations.

Do I have the courage to decline or face prolonged treatment?

This is a question you cannot answer until you have you answered the previous ones – and made your choice based on a firm understanding of your options.

It may help you to view your treatment as a short sprint rather than an endurance test if you remind yourself that you *always* have the right to withdraw from treatment at *any* stage. The only way to retain control over your life is to focus on what is best for you, whether you think the treatment is necessary and worthwhile, and what you are prepared to tolerate in order to survive. Your efforts to beat or live with your disease can only succeed if you, and all those caring for you, maintain this positive attitude.

The impact of fear

Previous experiences often determine the way we respond to things. It's highly likely that your fear of treatment and, by association, dread of doctors stems from painful and frightening childhood memories imprinted on you when you were vaccinated by the school nurse or doctor: the powerlessness you felt when you stood in line waiting your turn, the pain of the needle, your tears that were ignored.

Memories like these may explain why so many people avoid going to doctors even when their symptoms can no longer be ignored: the smoker's cough that won't go away, the lump that gets bigger and bigger, the pressing pains in the chest. Some people are afraid of having their worst fears confirmed, even though they are aware that early treatment usually means a better chance of success – so they ignore the messages their bodies are sending them.

The roots of your anxiety may be more recent – they may stem from an event that affected someone close to you, an article you read in a magazine, a dramatised television program you watched. If you've ever stood by someone fighting pain or clinging to life-supporting machines, you may fear going through the same experiences. Your fears may be sharpened if you've read stories about people being given incorrect diagnoses, treated for the wrong disease, having their X-rays mixed up with someone else's.

If the prospect of treatment strikes fear into your heart, you may be comforted to know that you are not alone. Most people are afraid of pain and other side effects, fears that are usually alleviated when they realise these effects can almost always be relieved and that treatment is not forever.

The sticky issue of alternative treatments

The word 'alternative' is widely used to describe any treatment that is not part of the established medical system of GPs, specialists, nurses and hospitals – but remember, the word is misleading if it makes you think that medicine offers no alternatives. In truth, medicine offers many choices, including the option of a second or third opinion.

Alternative treatments are normally used to treat back problems, headaches, arthritis, insomnia, structural pain in bones, cartilage, muscles and tendons. They involve acupuncture, chiropractic and homeopathic techniques, special diets, vitamins and trace-element supplements. These are all, essentially, lifestyle changes; while they make you feel better, more positive, more in control of your life, they are not the kind of therapeutic intervention you need when your life is on the line. They can be a valuable *complement* to medical treatments; and they can improve the quality of your life if you are absolutely certain there is nothing more that medicine can do for your particular condition, but they should never be used *instead* of medical treatment.

Almost everyone diagnosed with cancer is likely to face constant suggestions to try alternative treatments, mostly non-medical in nature. The pressure to take this path may be brought about by your own fears or the urgings of your family, friends and workmates who inundate you with tales of someone they know who was cured of cancer, for example, by eating nothing else except grapes, fasting, dieting, or introducing vitamins and nutrients into your diet. It's hard to fend off their pleas, especially when you put your own better judgement to one side because you don't want to hurt their feelings by not listening to them.

Many treatments for cancer are underpinned by the notion that cancer, ageing and death are unnatural and can, therefore, be eliminated forever. This belief is completely unrealistic. People get cancer even if they eat all the right foods, exercise regularly, are not overweight, neither smoke nor drink. In a normal frame of mind you may recognise this, but in the face of decreased life expectancy, you may be panicked into searching for someone who is willing to help you deny the seriousness, even the existence, of your condition.

In the face of being told by a doctor that there is nothing more that he can do for you, it's natural to look for someone who can offer you a miracle – and you will clutch at straws to find one. You may be drawn to treatments that help to give you back a sense of self-control, and submerge your fears of isolation, suffering and dying. If self-help programs give you the courage to face your treatment and improve your quality of life, they are worth pursuing, but I urge you to look elsewhere if the advocates of these programs disparage your doctor, ridicule medical treatments, and prevent you from obtaining a treatment that could reverse or halt the course of your cancer. You can easily commit errors of judgement you would not normally make when you're stressed out, up against a deadline, don't know what to do. It's hard to separate fact from fiction when what you hear is what you want to hear. You are highly exploitable when you are prepared to do anything to avoid pain and suffering, or to defy death.

There are some people who will tell you, or imply, that they can help you conquer cancer without medical treatment, that their therapies are more gentle, more effective, or both. I believe they are wrong. My own extensive experience with alternative therapies (see Chapter 1 for some of those I tried after my first cancer diagnosis) and the experience of every person I have counselled over the years confirms that these regimens are not capable of curing cancer on their own. Some alternative approaches, such as meditation, may improve the quality of your life and in conjunction with medical treatments may promote healing. Other approaches are less valuable.

Some reasons why you may be attracted to alternative therapies

1   You don't want to be seen by your family and friends as 'giving in' or 'letting down the side'. They want you to keep fighting. They may urge you to 'hang tough', 'fight it' – you fear rejection, even isolation, if you don't.

2   Your family and friends want you to try alternative treatments because they can't accept you told them you want to 'die with dignity'. You may want to be left alone, but your family won't give up.

3   You or your family may be persuaded that there is a conspiracy to deprive you of a cure for your cancer. (Why would anyone want to do such a thing? Conspiracy theories abound. Beware of them.)

4   You or your family may have been led to believe that alternative treatments produce no side effects. This is not true. As I explain later in this chapter, some of these treatments can be fatal.

If you are afraid of the side effects of medical treatment, the promise of a harmless treatment can be very seductive. Remember, though, that many treatments produce no side effects or quite mild ones. When I used 2-CDA to eradicate the last traces of my leukemia, the only side effect was an increased appetite. Reactions also vary between individuals. Even if you know someone who reacted badly to treatment, this does not mean you will.

Claims for alternative therapies
Most of the currently available alternative therapies have been around for decades – some since the last century – yet they are often offered as 'the latest advance' in the fight against cancer.

For as long as it is in vogue, each therapy has no rivals. People swear by it. After a while, its presumed effectiveness becomes diluted by reality, but then along comes another one, then another, and so on: hundreds and hundreds of them. To list a few and their originators:

1890s	Bacterial toxins	William Coley
1924	Essiac	Rene Caisse
1920s	Iscador	Rudolph Steiner
1920s	Live cell therapy	Paul Niehaus
1930s	Detoxification	Max Gerson
	Cancell	Jim Sheridan
1950s	Laetrile	various sources
1960s	Wheat Grass	Anne Wigmore
1970s	Germ cell therapy	Livingston-Wheeler
	High dose Vitamin C	Linus Pauling
1980s	Shark cartilage	Robert Langer
	Evening primrose oil	David Horrobin

If each new drug had been as successful as claimed, nothing would have taken its place and conventional medical treatment would have been discarded ages ago. But this has not happened. Instead, medical science continues to make exciting discoveries, many of which have already saved countless lives – mine included. It is important you are aware of these issues. Year in, year out, innumerable people waste precious time and hard-earned money pursuing false promises, false gods. I know all about this from my own experience and those of many people I have counselled. I caution you against them.

Alternative practitioners often claim that they, unlike doctors, treat the whole person and that doctors only treat presenting symptoms. There may be some validity in this claim when applied to general practitioners, but cancer and cardiac specialists invariably treat the whole person (their physical as well as their emotional states), and constantly recommend lifestyle changes to them to greatly improve their chances of recovery.

There are, undoubtedly, many alternative practitioners who believe in what they do, and do not seek to take advantage of you. I need hardly remind you that sincerity is a poor substitute for a successful outcome.

The outlook for many cancers is promising, particularly in the field of gene therapy. Early detection and gene screening continue to ensure that more effective and earlier treatment takes place – and early detection means better results.

The choice is yours

The number of alternative therapies promoted overtly and covertly to cure you of cancer are numerous and varied. We live, fortunately, in a society in which you can exercise freedom of choice. If none of the standard or non-standard medical treatments appeals to you or offers you grounds for optimism, it is your right to try anything you like to treat your cancer. No one has the right to prevent you. No one has the right to withhold information about treatments from you. You have to appreciate, though, that you must take responsibility for your decision.

This presents a dilemma to many people who try alternative therapies and are then compelled to return to their specialists in a last-ditch attempt to ease their symptoms, save their lives. They swallow copious amounts of 'immune-boosting' drugs, put their arms out for intravenous vitamins and cleansing agents, and place unusual instruments in a particular orifice to detoxify their bodies. Nothing works. Each story I know has been a personal tragedy, in most instances seriously affecting the family as well.

I understand this well. I also tried every available alternative treatment in an attempt to overcome my first cancer. Despite everything, I kept dying. When I had less than three months to live, medical science saved my life.

Questions to ask yourself about alternative therapies

The only way you can measure the value of any treatment is to compare its success rate against its failure rate, under the same conditions, treating the same disease, using the same methods. Conventional medical treatments are continually measured and assessed; alternative treatments are not.

If you are considering following an alternative therapy, I urge you and your family to consider these important questions before making a final decision.

☞ *Do I have to believe in the treatment before it can work?*

The advocates of many alternative therapies tell people not to embark on a nutritional therapy unless they firmly believe it will work for them.[3] This tactic lays the blame squarely on you should it fail – as it will if you have cancer. Many well-known psychiatric studies on cancer patients show that guilt is one of the most reliable symptoms of depression – and severe depression can make people suicidal.[4]

The proof of the pudding is in the eating, not in hoping it will taste good.

☞ *Has the treatment been tested in clinical trials?*

All clinical tests are reported in reputable scientific journals. Medical treatments are evaluated by other researchers and available for scrutiny in reputable scientific journals. This is not the case with alternative treatments. The results of medical trials can always be verified and replicated. You can find them in any medical library.

☞ *Does the treatment rely mostly on nutritional or diet therapy?*

While a high-fibre, low-fat diet, for example, might help prevent the recurrence of colorectal cancer and control coronary artery disease, there is no known dietary cure for cancer.

☞ *Is it claimed that the treatment being offered is harmless, painless or has no side effects?*

Most treatments that kill cancer cells properly will have side effects, although not everyone will experience them. Alternative treatments usually produce no side effects simply because they are ineffectual.

☞ *How long will the treatment take?*

Some medical treatments show results within a short space of time, they can be measured and predicted. Others take effect months later, so people who follow an alternative program might afterwards believe it was the alternative treatment that cured them.

☞ *How much will the treatment cost?*

This question demands one in return: why do the same people who complain about the high cost of medical treatment seldom complain about the cost of alternative treatments, often more expensive? Remember, the success factor in any treatment does not depend on how much you pay for it.

☞ *Do I really have cancer?*

If you have not been diagnosed by a cancer specialist, you may not have cancer at all or, if you do, it may be less serious than you thought. Moreover, many people who claim to have been cured by alternative treatments did not have cancer at all: the lump – palpable and uncomfortable as it was – was not malignant.

Three key questions to ask an alternative practitioner

Your failure to ask these questions could cost you your life.

1 How many patients with cancer have you successfully treated – and how many are in remission after five and ten years?
2 How many patients with *my* type of cancer have you successfully treated – and how many are in remission after five and ten years?
3 If I take this [vitamin C, for example] what percentage chance of recovery will you give me?

Ask for proof. If the alternative practitioner hesitates, tells you that not even a doctor would answer these questions, or that he or she has no records but they can help you anyway, back out the door – fast!

These are tough questions any successful cancer specialist would be willing to provide an answer for, with documentation to support their opinion.

Some consequences you may have to face if you forsake medical treatment

☞ Your symptoms will become progressively worse.
☞ You will waste valuable time in receiving treatment that may control your symptoms but do nothing to halt your disease.
☞ In rare cases, you may miss out on urgently needed treatment – if, for example, you have a tumor obstructing a bowel or a lung mass that hinders your breathing.
☞ You may forsake the opportunity to receive treatment that would allow you to spend precious time with your family and friends.
☞ You could be putting your health and even your life in jeopardy.

When drugs react with each other, they can become highly toxic and therefore dangerous. Not all alternative treatments are as harmless or as effective as claimed. For example, Vitamin C, in combination with certain chemotherapy drugs, can kill you. Laetrile (derived from apricot kernels which contain cyanide) and Iscador (derived from the mistletoe plant) have not only proved ineffective against cancer, they are lethal in large doses. Anything taken to excess can be dangerous. Increasing your vitamin intake – especially the fat-soluble vitamins A and D – can be highly toxic.

Various long-term studies were conducted in the USA, Finland and China among thousands of smokers, non-smokers and asbestos workers who were given supplements to test if high doses of beta-carotene and vitamins A and E could protect them against lung cancer. The studies were halted when they found that smokers who took the vitamins were at *increased* risk compared with those who did not.[5]

Your body only absorbs what it needs and secretes the rest. Someone once said that the best thing about vitamins is that they produce very expensive urine. However, if you're still tempted to take vitamins and dietary supplements, tell your cancer specialist – just to be safe.

☞   You may give credit for your recovery to someone who doesn't deserve it.

In one particular case, a doctor of Chinese medicine told a woman I was counselling that he thought it was a good idea for her to continue with chemotherapy because, 'It will help *my* herbs get rid of your cancer.'

Facts and myths about cancer
THE MYTHS
1   If you don't get cancer, you'll live to a ripe old age.
2   Cancer is always fatal.
3   Cancer is always exhausting.
4   No one ever fully recovers from cancer.
5   Cancer is catching.
6   If a tumor is exposed to air it will spread.
7   Death from cancer is always painful.
8   Cancer always destroys your quality of life.

9   People with cancer look different.
10   You are to blame for your disease.

THE FACTS ABOUT CANCER

All of the above ten statements are wrong. What is firmly established is that medicine has made some spectacular gains over the past 60 years, yet in the world's richer countries one person in three will develop cancer and about one in four will die of it; in the USA one in three people will be diagnosed with cancer, and one in five will die from it. According to the World Health Organisation, about one-half of all cancers occur in the most industrialised one-fifth of the world's population.[6] The incidence of most diseases is on the decline, yet cancer is still on the increase and is, after coronary artery diseases, the second most common cause of death in most First World countries. On present trends, cancer will surpass heart disease as the number one cause of death in the twenty-first century. In Japan, it is already.[7]

These facts need to be viewed in the light of the World Health Organisation Report, 1997, *'Conquering Suffering, Enriching Humanity'*, which states that 'dramatic increases in life expectancy, combined with profound changes in lifestyles, will lead to global epidemics of cancer and other chronic diseases in the next two decades.' The report confirms that the incidence of cancer will increase in direct proportion to the increased life expectancy of the population. The older you get, the more likely you are to get cancer or some other degenerative disease. We cannot avoid the ageing process.

The World Health Organisation report confirms an earlier one conducted by the Australian Institute of Health and Welfare covering the period 1989-90. It noted that by the age of 75, one in three Australian men and one in four women get cancer; overall, 24 per cent of men and 22 per cent of women will die of it. Cancer is the only major cause of death that continues to rise, *yet more people die from causes other than cancer.*[8]

There are well over 100 different types of cancer and, because no two people are alike, it is most unlikely that one treatment will be found to deal with them all. After decades of research costing billions of dollars the nature of cancer is now more clearly understood than ever before, and yet this has not led to a total solution for 'the problem of cancer'. The 'magic bullet' for which scientists have been searching may be as elusive and unfathomable as the Loch Ness Monster. Even so, largely due to improved diagnostic procedures, almost half of everyone diagnosed with cancer will either be cured or go into remission. According to the National Cancer Institute in the USA, in 1996 over eight million Americans and 17.9 million people worldwide had a history of cancer. According to the Anti-Cancer Council of Victoria, the figure for Australia is around half a million, not including non-melanocytic (skin) cancers. It is also true that there are more treatments available for most types of cancer than for other life-threatening diseases.

The case for conventional treatment

If you are still concerned that medical treatment will be worse than the disease, here are some points for you to bear in mind:

- Medical treatments often cause significant side effects and varying degrees of discomfort, but these are relatively minor when compared to the often uncontrollable, unpleasant, painful and life-threatening effects of cancer if you *don't* have treatment.
- Most cancers detected at an early stage are potentially curable. Medical testing procedures have enabled doctors to detect many cancers early enough for them to be successfully treated.
- There is no type of cancer from which no one has recovered.
- Many more cancers are treatable today than they were even ten years ago. Cancer is the most curable of all chronic diseases.[9] Over half the people treated with conventional medicine will still be alive five years after their diagnosis.[10]
- Nearly half the people treated for cancer *never* require any further treatment; some cancers are easy to cure, some are not.[11] Many people live with cancer in the same way others live with diabetes. In my own case, I injected myself with interferon three times a week for almost four years before I found the drug that wiped out the last traces of my leukemia in one blow.
- The side effects of most treatments can be controlled or treated.

☞ Your doctor can offer you proven and documented evidence from around the world about the successes and failures of conventional medical treatments. If statistics exist for alternative treatments, they are unpublished, unverified and unproven.

Take a little time

Try to strike a balance between taking too long and acting too hastily to make a decision about treatment. If your symptoms don't bother you, you have a busy work schedule, or your doctor says, 'Let's wait and see,' you may be tempted to procrastinate. Remaining undecided for too long can put you at serious risk. As I will explain in more detail in the following chapter, cancer cells grow at a geometric rate: 2, 4, 8, 16, 32, etc. It is much easier to treat cancer before it spreads. On the other hand, it's unlikely that a few days will be critical – and they may make all the difference.

I believe it is what we still hope for and expect from life that can make the difference between a successful and an unsuccessful treatment. At the same time, it would be highly unusual if you weren't filled with doubts about your ability to cope. You have to take risks, but consider them as coolly and as rationally as possible – no mean feat when you feel as if you're looking down the barrel of a gun, as I was when I was diagnosed with lung cancer.

The doctors wanted to operate on me immediately. I wanted to understand more about lung cancers before I committed myself to surgery. In the week I took to research the subject, consider my treatment options, examine other possibilities if any, and come to terms with a second diagnosis of cancer, I found the most experienced and skilled surgeons and anaesthetist, established what was possible and what wasn't, and made out a living will in case I became unable to make my own decisions.

Quality of life

Over the past half-century or so, there has been amazing progress in the treatment of certain diseases, in easing pain, prolonging life; but the same medical technology that can keep you from dying can often keep you from living. If you are kept alive through life-support systems but are unable to enjoy some activity – physical or mental – you may well ask, 'Is life worth living?'

We take good health for granted until we become ill and face the dilemma: do we become victims of our disease or prisoners of technology? We have to consider how far we are prepared to go in letting our doctors treat us, what sacrifices we are ready to make, how long we are prepared to face treatments and their side effects. The prize we seek is life, but at what price? To live as if we were vegetables attached to a hydroponic feeding system?

Your doctor's idea of what 'success' means may not be the same as yours, so it is essential to discuss this candidly with your doctor, and consider carefully how far you want him to go in maintaining your vital functions if this means

(a)   remaining permanently unconscious; or

(b)   being conscious but confined to bed; or

(c)   being conscious but unable to live your life as you would want to live it; or

(d)   being conscious but indefinitely dependent upon family and friends.

People often tell me that if they were given the choice, they would be prepared to trade survival time in favour of quality of life. Not one has said they want to linger on in an unconscious or semi-conscious state; all maintain they want to retain self-respect, would rather die with dignity than live every day in fear.

I am also aware that many people move the goalposts in determining their quality of life, as Alan did, a friend of mine who suffered the progressively crippling motor neurone disease, ALS, amylotrophic lateral sclerosis.

Shortly after he was diagnosed, and aware that his life-span would be dramatically reduced, Alan said he did not want to live if he could no longer walk; when he could no longer walk, he chose his inability to manage his personal hygiene as his deadline; when he had to rely on 24-hour nursing care, he set inability to speak as his endpoint. Two years after his diagnosis, and when he was no longer able to speak, he developed pneumonia, refused to be placed on a respirator, and chose to die.

Sexual potency makes an interesting marker of 'quality of life', for men at least. Aware that sexual potency is intimately linked to our life force, the authors of one study focused on discovering how men would respond to the choice between survival on one hand and maintaining sexual potency on the other if they underwent surgery for prostate cancer.

Their results showed that in order to maintain sexual potency, 32 per cent were unwilling to trade off any survival, but 68 per cent were willing to trade off a 10 per cent or greater advantage over a five-year period. The basis of this trial was that while surgery for prostate cancer offers a higher survival rate (90 per cent at five years), it also produces a 90-100 per cent rate of sexual impotency. Radiotherapy, the alternative, produces a 20-50 per cent rate of impotency, but the survival rate is much lower. The authors of the study wrote that

> Patients should be permitted to choose medical treatments according to their own values, beliefs, preferences and life goals. In this way, we empower patients and put into operation the concept of autonomy. People can exercise this right to choose only if their physician informs them of options in treatments. [12]

Whichever treatment program you and your doctor agree upon, you both need to appreciate that quality of life is not a mere rating of the status of your health, nor is it determined by an increase in survival time. Unless you are in agreement on the matter, your doctor's values should play no role in deciding whether the often-unpleasant side effects of treatment are worth it or not. Moreover, you should bear no resentment if you are not cured or do not have the outcome you hoped for. In other words, a good attitude does affect the quality of life but should not be expected to affect the quantity of life.

Bear in mind that alternative therapists do not have the sole franchise on 'quality of life'. People who shun conventional treatment in favour of alternative treatments often end up losing more quality of life. From my experience, quality of life comes when you are *not* in pain, are *not* bleeding uncontrollably, have support, are *not* afraid, are in control of your bodily functions. Quality of life comes when you are able to do what you want to do, when you feel that life still holds promise.

Why treatment has to stop

The aim of medical technology is to provide you with temporary support until your body can take over its previous functions – i.e. until you are restored to health and able to lead a normal life.

Sometimes this has to take place in stages. For example, the treatment for your particular cancer may involve two periods of chemotherapy or radiotherapy each lasting ten days, with a three-week break in between. The interval is prescribed for one good reason: normal cells could not withstand such relentless treatment without time to recover.

Once this intensive treatment is over, you may go into maintenance therapy, often for a lifetime (as with asthma and diabetes). Some cancer treatments, particularly those involving the use of hormones, steroids and biological agents, follow this pattern.

Your doctor should tell you precisely how long your treatment will last and how frequently it will be administered. If he hasn't, you must ask. It is vital that you and your family know this, or else you're all likely to be angered and distressed when your treatment is discontinued. Instead of seeing this as a sign that your doctor is giving up on you, see it for what it is:

☞ time for your treatment to take effect and time for your body to recover;

☞ time and the opportunity for you to take responsibility for your own healing; and

☞ time to change your view of yourself from that of a patient with a plastic tag around your wrist to a person with a potentially new lease of life, as a survivor aware that healing is possible even when a cure is not.

What is healing?

Of course you want to be cured, restored to health. Regaining your health, however, is not an end in itself, but a means to an end: to enable you to seek the answers to the meaning of life while doing something purposeful and worthwhile with it. Wholeness ('healing', 'wholeness' and 'health' have the same root) occurs when you bring these elements together.

The miracle of healing occurs when you realise that there may be no rational answer to your illness, choose to take responsibility for your own care, give yourself over to a power greater than yourself.

Healing is the natural effect of marshalling your own inner resources when you choose to be a survivor. Healing is an internal process, doesn't depend on anything outside of yourself. Healing begins when you no longer see your disease as an alien force to be conquered at all costs, but rather as a symbol of the old self you need to relinquish in order to start life anew. It cannot begin as long as you want life to return to the way it was before your diagnosis.

The healing journey starts when you accept that change is in the natural order of things, that the only way to go is forward, that to cling to your old ways is likely to confirm the ancient Chinese proverb, 'Changelessness is death.'

Healing happens when you finally shift the focus away from your intellect and into your heart – when you 'take heart', acquiesce in the mystery of life. It is then that you are granted the reprieve – and the energy – to discover that there are some immutable forces at work, the nature of which we can only guess; and that death, like life, cannot be avoided. Healing then becomes soundness of body, mind and spirit.

Can you protect yourself against cancer?

According to the World Health Organisation Report, 1990,[13] the precise *cause* of a type of cancer cannot be identified unless it produces the same effect in *all* people. The most clearly established cancer-causing agent is tobacco smoking, whether chewed or snuffed or smoked as cigarettes, pipes or cigars.

It is far easier to estimate the risks of cancer for whole populations. This is based on measuring the number of new cases of cancer (the incidence) that occur in a defined population, and the rate at which they occur over a given period of time.

☞ Age is the most powerful predictor of cancer (the longer you live, the higher the risk), but its effects vary in different countries.

☞ Oddly enough, your religion can make a difference, too. Cancer of the penis is rare among Jewish males who are circumcised at birth, and Jewish women seldom get uterine cervix cancer. In the USA, Mormons and Seventh-Day

Adventists abstain from smoking and drinking, and so infrequently get the types of cancers caused by these agents.[14]

☞ Your job can put you at risk, especially if you are exposed to well-known *carcinogens*, agents that cause cancer, particularly asbestos (higher in those who smoke), benzene, formaldehyde, diesel exhaust, hair dyes, pesticides, radiation, and radon (mostly affecting miners).

☞ Cancer treatments, including radiation and drugs, can also increase cancer risk, and the risk is varied. Those, for example, who have been treated with a combination of drugs for Hodgkin's lymphoma are at slightly higher risk of acute leukemia or, more rarely, bladder cancer. Tamoxifen, used to treat breast cancer, has been reported to cause the occasional case of endometrial cancer. In both these cases, people usually feel the advantages far outweigh the risk. (Oral contraceptives have been implicated in the risk of pre-menopausal breast and some types of liver cancer, yet they reduce the risk of ovarian and endometrial and, it is suspected, bowel and rectal cancer, as well.)

☞ Bacteria have also been implicated in certain cancers, in particular *Helicobacter pylori*, known to cause cancer of the stomach in humans.[15] This condition is now highly treatable through the use of antibiotics.

☞ Anything that grows on food is of concern. Aflotoxin, a mould found on peanuts, has been implicated in some cancers in developing countries.

☞ Excessive exposure to the sun's ultraviolet rays is the main cause of non-melanoma skin cancer, the most common of all cancers, and malignant melanoma, which is far more serious.

☞ Ionising radiation from atomic blasts and radiation, as well as from certain fertilisers, building materials and X-rays, can cause leukemia, thyroid and skin cancer.

☞ Genetic inheritance can predispose people to certain cancers. There is a two to four times higher rate of cancers of the stomach, breast, large intestine, uterus and lung in relatives of people who have had cancer, and this link has also been noted in leukemia, brain tumors in children, and sarcomas.

☞ Genital herpes in women gives rise to a higher incidence of cancer of the cervix of the uterus, while stomach cancer is five times higher in people with pernicious anaemia and associated gastritis.

☞ The country in which you live and its associated lifestyles is a strong indicator of certain types of cancer. San Francisco has the highest rate of breast cancer, Nowy Sacz in Poland has the lowest; North America, Europe, Japan, Australia and Russia have the highest rates of lung cancer, India and Dakar (Africa) the lowest.

☞ Poverty and malnutrition dramatically increase the incidence of oral and esophageal cancer.

☞ The effects of diet or the way food is prepared are less clear. There would appear to be more of a link with what is *not* in your diet than what is. There is evidence to suggest that naturally occurring substances – most of which are vegetable-based – can actually *prevent* cancer.[16] The buzz words for many years were 'beta carotene' and 'vitamin A', but world studies on these substances were halted when it was found they actually increased the risk of cancer. [17]

In general, it is difficult to measure diet as a risk factor for cancer in a scientific way that precludes other factors. You can help to *reduce the risk* of getting it by making changes to your lifestyle – but there are no guarantees.

So what can you do?

To lower your risk of getting cancer, the suggestions below are based on the guidelines laid down by the American Institute for Cancer Research, the Harvard Center for Cancer Prevention, and the Peter MacCallum Cancer Institute, Australia.

SMOKING, ALCOHOL, DIET

If you smoke, stop. If you're not a smoker, don't start. Smoking is a life-shortening habit.

Drink alcohol only in moderation, if at all. Even two drinks a day has been associated with an increased risk of breast cancer. Smoking *and* drinking sharply increase the risk of cancers of the lung, upper respiratory and digestive tract; even in smaller quantities, they can lead to breast and colorectal cancer.

Eating a healthier diet is likely to help protect you not only against cancer, but also against heart disease, stroke and a variety of other health problems.

- Limit your intake of salt, a likely cause of stomach cancer. Nitrates and nitrites – used as a preservative in meats and other cured products, and sometimes present in bacon, cheeses and beer – have also been linked to stomach and esophageal cancer.

- Increase your consumption of fruits, vegetables and whole grains. An increase in these foods (as well as bread, rice, cereal, beans and pasta) can significantly reduce the risk of respiratory and gastro-intestinal cancer, particularly colon cancer.

- Avoid burnt food; high temperatures can generate lots of chemicals which may cause cancer.

- Take half an aspirin a day with food. Apart from lowering the risk of a heart attack or stroke, it can help lower the likelihood of getting bowel cancer.

- Don't overeat. Obesity is an important cause of endometrial cancer, and weakly linked to breast cancer in post-menopausal women. Obesity also increases the risk of cancers of the colon, gall bladder and kidneys.

SCREENING AND TESTING

Early detection of cancer can mean the difference between life and death from many cancers. In general, men and women over 40, especially those in a high-risk category, should have annual cancer-related physical check-ups by a cancer specialist.

- To test for cervical cancer, women should have regular pap smears. At the same time, a pelvic examination can test for uterine and endometrial cancers.

- To test for breast cancer, women should routinely examine their breasts for lumps. If they are over 50 and have a family history of breast cancer, they should have a mammogram annually.

☞ Men should learn to examine their testicles for unusual lumps to test for testicular cancer.

☞ If you're a man over 50, it is advisable to have a PSA test and digital rectal examination annually to test for prostate cancer.

☞ Men and women over 40 should have digital rectal examinations and stool tests annually to check for colorectal cancers.

☞ Keep an eye on any sore that does not heal or for changes to moles; and nominate someone in your family to watch your back regularly.

EXERCISE

Exercise has been directly linked to lowering the risk for certain types of cancer, such as cancer of the colon, rectum, prostate, endometrium, breast and kidney, and also helps reduce the risk for heart disease. Obesity can predispose you to heart attacks, stroke, diabetes, arthritis, liver and gall bladder disease, and cancer of the gastro-intestinal tract.

Twenty to 30 minutes of moderate exercise most days of the week is a good idea.

STAY OUT OF THE SUN

In Australia, two out of three people will have at least one skin cancer by the time they are 74. Getting burnt by the sun in childhood or early adolescence presents a higher risk of developing melanoma later in life (it can often take up to 20 years for cancer to develop).

There is clear evidence that sailors and people who work outdoors are more at risk of developing lip cancer than of melanoma; lighter-skinned people are at higher risk than dark-skinned people. Take precautions. If you have to go out in the sun, cover yourself; desert dwellers do.

AVOID RADIATION

Radiation risk refers to exposure to electromagnetic fields around power cables, and from X-rays, radon, fluorescent lighting, and radiotherapy treatment. With the exception of radiotherapy and X-rays which present relatively higher risks, the evidence of danger from the others is scant. In the early days, microwave ovens and television sets were considered hazardous, but are now safe.

- ☞ Don't have dental X-rays more than once every two years.
- ☞ Keep medical exposure to X-rays to a minimum – especially if you're pregnant.
- ☞ Try to live away from nuclear plants.

Evidence on radiation risk is always changing. People most at risk appear to be power-station and nuclear-plant workers, linesmen, telecommunication, radio and television repairmen.[18]

...AND FINALLY...

It is my view that the incidence of cancer will decrease over time as we adapt to the environmental hazards to which we are presently so susceptible. The by-products of the industrial revolution are relatively new on the time-scale of man's existence. I believe that, in the distant future, mankind will become inured to the toxic and carcinogenic substances in the environment.

There are, however, some sensible things you can do. You can get more sleep, and stop abusing your body. You can't change your parents, so you're stuck with your genes, but this doesn't mean you will get cancer even if they did. And even if you do, you can still survive it. I believe survivors are people who understand what is happening to them, face up to the challenge of a life-threatening disease, establish a therapeutic partnership with a cancer specialist, and discover the wisdom of God woven into the fabric of their body and soul.

seven

treatment options

&

'The rules of the game do not require us to win
at all costs, but they do demand that we
never give up the fight.'

VIKTOR FRANKL

So what are your treatment options? You are probably familiar with
the more well-known medical treatments for cancer such as surgery,
chemotherapy, radiotherapy and hormone therapy. As I will explain
in this chapter, there are other options, some quite novel, which hold
great promise for the future.

But before you read about these, it is important for you to understand some basic facts.

How cells work

All living things are made up of cells. Inside each of these cells are
certain molecules – *genes* – which consist of a stretch of Deoxyribo-
Nucleic Acid (DNA) and which not only control the function of
cells, but contain all the inherited information that makes you the
individual you are.

Every cell in your body grows by dividing itself into two identical
cells. In the process of division, each daughter cell receives an identical copy of its mother cell's DNA.

DNA is locked away inside the nucleus, or core, of each cell, and
cannot put its instructions into practice without help. The messenger
it uses to carry out its commands is a flexible one-strand molecule
called RiboNucleic Acid – RNA.

To ensure there is no breakdown in communications, DNA uses
one of its relatively rigid double helix strands (which look like a

twisted stepladder) as a template to copy, or transcribe, the information it wants to send onto an RNA strand. The RNA then relays these instructions to the cell's minute protein-making factories called *ribosomes,* which churn out the vital proteins necessary to create new cells and ensure the smooth operation of all those functions necessary to keep us alive. For example, some proteins such as collagen and keratin hold our tissues and bodies in shape. Proteins such as insulin act as messengers between cells, while hemoglobin carries oxygen around our body. Moreover, in a process that is the very miracle of life, from the moment a sperm and an ovum get together, the resultant embryo knows what to become or, as the case may be, what *not* to become. This process is called *differentiation.* Some cells become various parts of the body – legs, arms, body, head. Other cells become various organs such as the heart, lung, liver, kidney and spleen. Some cells produce the pigment in your skin, others become the pathways along which messages are sent from your brain to various parts of your body. A muscle cell, for instance, cannot perform the function of a nerve cell, a blood cell cannot take the place of an acid-producing cell.

Some cells stop growing when we become adults, others retain their ability to divide so that they can replace those cells which wear out and die. Mature red blood cells, for example, cannot reproduce themselves. As they wear out or are lost through bleeding, they are replaced in the bone marrow via undifferentiated cells, sometimes known as mother cells. Cells in your skin, hair, digestive system and liver are constantly replacing themselves. Each time a cell divides, it replaces its DNA, and any mistakes which are made in the process are quickly corrected. Occasionally, however, a defective cell continues to divide and replicate its defective DNA. This is what happens when a mutation takes place. Sometimes, but not always, it can have serious results. For example, faulty insulin leads to diabetes, faulty hemoglobin to anaemia.

What is cancer?

Cancer cells are not foreign cells, but are part of our own bodies. Cancer occurs when genes go haywire and cells, instead of maintaining an orderly pattern of cell growth, begin to grow rapidly, abnormally, and without restraint. When normal cells become cancerous, they change their appearance and their behaviour, lose their ability to differentiate, and start dividing out of control. Cancer cells grow geometrically: 2 becomes 4, then 16, then 32 and so on. The smallest number of cancer cells that can be detected by feel, X-ray, scan or mammogram is 10^9 – a thousand million cells.

In the normal process of cell division, differentiated cells are repaired and renewed by other differentiated cells. For example, if you break a bone, 'bone' cells will race to the injured site and restore the bone to its original pre-designed shape. When they have done their job, they stop. Cancer cells don't know when to stop. If left unchecked, they will move out of their original site and invade and destroy surrounding tissues. The word 'cancer' is derived from the Greek word for crab, and describes the pincer-like invasion of normal cells by cancerous cells. These can be a mixture of types: tumors are not always composed only of tumor cells, but are often a mixture of normal blood cells, immune-system cells, connective-tissue cells and so on.

On the whole, genes aren't often inherited in an already mutated form, but when this does occur, it causes diseases such as sickle-cell anaemia, hemophilia, Tay-Sachs disease, Huntingdon's chorea. External factors, such as tobacco smoke or high doses of radiation, sunlight and viruses can also cause genes to mutate. When genes are thrown into disorder because the molecular structure of the DNA has been mutated, this can cause the affected cells to become cancerous.

Anything that damages genes can cause cancer. Whether it does depends on individual differences, the environment in which you live, your body's response, your genetic make-up, or perhaps some event affecting your genes after your birth. Inherited cancers are the rarest of all, yet some people carry genes that make people susceptible to cancer-causing agents. Where you live and your lifestyle can also cause cancer. For example, Australia has the highest rate of skin cancer; worldwide, smoking accounts for 30 per cent of all cancers, while obesity, high salt intake, poor nutrition and lack of exercise are responsible for 35 per cent of all cancer cases.[1]

Cancer is not a single disease, but rather the generic name used for more than 100 diseases, all having in common the uncontrolled reproduction of abnormal cells. We are all prone to what Shakespeare says are 'the thousand natural shocks that flesh is heir to'.

What is neoplasia?

Neoplasia means 'new growth'. It refers to cells which grow abnormally and excessively without being influenced by the body's normal control mechanisms. A neoplasm can be either benign or malignant.

Benign and malignant growths can be hard to distinguish, so tests are essential in order to determine the difference between them before any treatment can begin.

Benign growths, by definition, do not metastasise (see below), but can often be just as dangerous as malignant ones if, for example, they grow larger and obstruct a blood vessel or an airway.

What is malignancy?

Cancer cells are termed malignant if they have four specific features:

1   POOR DIFFERENTIATION

As described earlier, differentiation refers to the ability of cells to develop specific and highly individualised functions whereby cells become distinguished from each other.

In neoplasia, the new cells arise from previously 'normal-looking' cells. They may either resemble the normal cells from which they arose, or they may take on a completely new appearance in which case they are said to be 'poorly differentiated'. They often look bizarre.

2   RAPID GROWTH RATE

In general, benign tumors grow slowly and malignant ones grow quickly. There are, as always, exceptions to the rule. The same tumor may also grow at different rates and different times. Another general rule is that rapidly growing tumors are often composed of poorly differentiated cells.

3   LOCAL INVASION

Local invasion is the process by which tumors can infiltrate, invade or destroy surrounding healthy tissues as they grow larger. Local invasion and metastases (see below) are key features of malignant tumors.

4   METASTASIS AND SECONDARIES

Some cancer cells may detach themselves from their original site, known as the primary site, and invade blood vessels, nerve sheaths and lymphatic tissue. The process whereby malignant cells locate themselves elsewhere in the body away from their original site is called *metastasis*. The result of this renegade activity are secondary growths, commonly known as *secondaries* (metastases).

Unlike invasion, in metastasis there is no continuous pathway of malignant cells from the original site. Metastatic cancer cells are virtually identical in appearance and behaviour to the original tumor. For example, a breast cancer which has metastasised to the lymph nodes would be called 'lymphatic metastasis from a primary breast cancer' and not 'a cancer of the lymph glands'. In much the same manner, colon cancer which has metastasised to the liver is not called liver cancer.[2]

Research indicates there may be some credibility to the tumor dormancy concept: the hypothesis that some primary tumors actually suppress secondary tumors, i.e. the secondaries remain dormant until the primary tumor is removed, at which point they erupt.[3]

What is carcinoma?

Cancers originating in those cells which line an organ such as the larynx, lung, stomach and intestines are called *carcinomas*.

Skin cancer is also a carcinoma, because it occurs in the body's 'lining', the skin.

'Adeno' refers to the cells lining any gland, including the lung and breast, so an *adeno-carcinoma* refers to cancer of these cells.

A *squamous cell carcinoma* is a specific type of lung cancer – 'squamous' referring to the large, flat cells which line the bronchial tubes.

What is sarcoma?

Sarcoma is cancer of soft or connective tissues such as muscles, nerves, tendons, blood vessels, cartilage and bones.

Sarcomas have been distinguished from carcinomas since the time of Hippocrates. The word sarcoma is derived from the Greek root *sarc* (flesh) in contrast to 'crablike' carcinomas. The word 'sarcasm', or a flesh-tearing criticism, is derived from the same root.

What is melanoma?

Cancer of the pigment-producing cells in the skin is called *melanoma*.

What is leukemia and myeloma?

In adults, new white blood cells are formed in the marrow of membranous bones such as the spine, sternum, ribs and pelvis. Cancer of these cells is referred to as *leukemia*.

Myelomas are cancers of certain types of white cells which produce antibodies. The chief difference between them is that in leukemia, cancer cells are released into the blood; in myeloma, most of them remain in the bone.

What is lymphoma?

Cancer of the lymphatic system is called *lymphoma*.

The lymphatic system is a circulation system, much like the blood system. It performs two major functions. It drains off all excess fluid from tissues, and as part of our body's immune system, it recognises foreign substances such as germs and traps them in its glands, or nodes, where they can be destroyed by white blood cells. Although they are concentrated in the neck, groin and armpits, lymph nodes are found all over the body.

What is the difference between remission, response and cure?

If you understand these terms clearly, there will be less chance of a disjunction between what your doctors says and what you think he means.

A *complete response* or *complete remission* means there is no more evidence of your cancer.

A *partial response* or *partial remission* is when your cancer cells have shrunk to less than 50 per cent of their original size and there is significant relief from your symptoms; it means there is a good chance you will live longer.

A *disease-free survival* means the time between a complete remission and the recurrence of cancer.

Duration of response means the time between achieving a remission to the time the cancer starts growing again.

A *cure* is more difficult to define. Because it is, doctors tend to hide behind words such as 'partial remission' or 'complete remission'.

People often make the mistake of believing that if their doctor tells them their cancer is 'inoperable' then it is 'incurable'. This is not so. Your cancer may not be able to be treated surgically at this point in time, but chemotherapy and radiotherapy can be used to shrink it so it can be surgically removed later.

If you consider a cure to mean that you no longer have any of the symptoms of your disease, the obvious question this raises is, 'How long must you be symptom-free to be considered cured?' I think the only way you can honestly use the word 'cure' is when you mean that by the time you eventually die you have not experienced any more symptoms of your cancer.

Pre-treatment tests

In order to provide you with the most effective treatment with the least possible number of side effects, your doctor has to establish some baseline measurements about you and your cancer, where it is located, if it has spread, and where. In some cases you may need to have several different tests so your doctor can be sure.

These tests are also important so that the effectiveness of your treatment can be measured, in terms of your cancer and your general health. You should ask your doctor to tell you which tests he will ask you to have.

Here is a short summary of some of the more basic ones he will use.

BLOOD TEST

Blood tests can tell your doctor just about everything about you – if you have an infection or a disease, if you have enough oxygen in your blood, and if your blood can clot, if there are problems with your liver, your kidneys, and your immune system. The state of every organ in your body can be read in a blood test.

It can also tell your doctor if the treatment has worked.

ULTRASONOGRAPHY

Just as submarines use sonar to locate enemy submarines, so ultrasound can enable your doctor to detect areas of abnormal density. In this way, he can measure the shape and size of a cancer, also tell if it is solid or not. Ultrasound can even spot the difference between a cyst and a cancer.

Nuclear medicine

Radioactive substances, called radionuclides, can be injected into you and will be taken up to different extents by different tissues and organs. A scanner is then passed over you, and the intensity of the emissions fed into a computer. The image it constructs can tell your doctor not only about the position of a cancer, but whether the organ or tissue it has affected is functioning properly.

Radionuclides can also be given by mouth, are not toxic, and are significantly lower in radiation than alternative X-ray techniques.

A PET (Positron Emission Tomography) scan is the most sensitive device available to nuclear medicine. Positrons are sub-atomic particles that travel for a few millimetres in tissue and are used in conjunction with radionuclides to pick up highlighted cancers which might otherwise be obscured by an organ.

Scanning
(a)   X-rays are electromagnetic waves that are passed through you onto a photographic plate. Your bones are denser than your muscles and fat, so X-rays reaching the film after passing through bone will expose the film less than those passing through soft tissue. Just as X-ray pictures show white bones on a black background, so solid tumors also show up clearly.
(b)   CAT (Computer Aided Tomography) scans pass narrow X-ray beams through your body from different angles to produce a series of cross-section images. CAT scans provide clearer, more highly defined pictures, a particularly useful characteristic in detecting tumors in soft tissue. CAT scans are often referred to as CT (Computerised Tomography) scans.
(c)   MRI (Magnetic Resonance Imaging) scans also provide cross-sections of your internal organs, but the process is much safer, as no X-rays are used.

The theory behind MRI is quite simple: hydrogen atoms in a powerful and stationary magnetic field absorb radio waves of a particular frequency. Strong magnets surrounding your body are turned on and off in succession. Turned on, they cause the hydrogen atoms to absorb these waves; turned off, the hydrogen atoms re-emit the energy they have absorbed, which is then fed into a computer to create a clear cross-section image.

MRI is the preferred, but costlier, method of testing because of its greater sensitivity and lack of radiation. As with CT scans, MRI testing requires an injection of a dye that highlights each organ. MRI scans tend to take better pictures of thin people, CAT scans better ones of fat people.

Endoscopy

In recent years, advances in fibre-optic technology have proved invaluable in locating tumors in the bowel, bronchial tubes, lung, and pancreatic ducts.

Your treatment choices: surgery

Surgery is the oldest and most clear-cut of all therapies. Current estimates place the cure rate of surgery on its own at over 60 per cent.[4] The aim of surgery, in most cases, is to remove the entire tumor *before it has spread.*

Surgery may be used to remove only a part of the tumor if the tumor is too large, inaccessible or dangerously located; chemotherapy or radiotherapy might then be used to attack the remaining cancer. In some cases, the entire tumor may be removed to improve the effects of radiotherapy or chemotherapy. Even when the outlook for a cure is poor, surgery is often used to alleviate pain or relieve the obstruction of hollow organs such as the stomach.

Sometimes cancers which are still small or at an early stage can be eliminated by surgery alone. If you have the slightest doubt that your cancer has spread, even though your surgeon said, 'I got it all,' bear in mind that one million cancer cells can fit on the head of a pin, one thousand million cancer cells are the size of a pea, so they can travel easily and swiftly through the blood stream or lymph system. Your peace of mind is as important to your recovery as surgery. Consult an oncologist and make sure you have all your bases covered.

SIDE EFFECTS OF SURGERY

The most usual consequence of any surgery is pain, frequently and often successfully controlled with a whole range of drugs, with low-dose morphine or opiates reserved for severe pain.

The more obvious long-term side effect of surgery is the loss of a part of your body. Most people come to terms with this eventually when they consider what the alternative might have been. Please read the following chapter for more details about pain control and ways of coping with physical and sexual problems.

Chemotherapy

Chemotherapy simply means treatment with drugs. When your doctor treats your sore throat with an antibiotic, he uses a drug to attack and kill germs. Chemotherapy is the use of *cytotoxic* drugs – that is, drugs that have the ability to kill cells. There are over 40 of these proven drugs currently in use on their own or in combination with others. Chemotherapy is used to treat localised as well as metastasised tumors. It is often used on its own, but can be used to shrink tumors so they can more easily be treated with radiotherapy, or removed by surgery.

Chemotherapy is also used to boost the effects of radiotherapy. Used in this way it is called additional chemotherapy or, as doctors and nurses say, *adjuvant* chemotherapy.

As with surgery, if chemotherapy cannot be used to overcome your cancer, it *can* be used as a palliative to relieve your symptoms, reduce your pain and discomfort – to help you feel as well as possible.

People often assume that if chemotherapy offers little chance of success in treating their particular cancer, there are no other options. If your cancer falls into this category, you still have other options – these are discussed later in this chapter.

HOW DOES CHEMOTHERAPY WORK?

The aim of chemotherapy is to disrupt the actual process of cell division – i.e. prevent the production of daughter cells. It does this either by interfering with, and preventing, DNA production, or by depriving cancer cells of the proteins they need in order to grow.

Cancer cells often divide faster than normal cells, which makes them more susceptible to drugs that attack cells in the process of dividing. However, the drugs can't tell the difference between a dividing cancer cell and a dividing normal cell, so the tissues which normally contain rapidly dividing cells – such as those in your hair follicles and those lining the intestine – are also likely to be affected. This explains why these drugs cause side effects such as baldness and diarrhoea.

Cancer cells do not all divide at the same rate or at the same time, so your doctor may choose to give you a 'cocktail' of drugs that act at different rates to take this into account. Results are often more spectacular than if you were given a single drug.

Even if it cannot cure your cancer, chemotherapy can be used to shrink your cancer, relieve pain or bleeding, slow the cancer's growth. As a general rule, chemotherapy is used to treat cancers that have spread, radiotherapy to treat cancers that have not spread. You should discuss with your doctor what he intends to achieve with this choice of therapy: a complete response, a partial response, or relief from your symptoms. Also ask for an explanation of the side effects and how these will be treated.

THE NOT-SO-GOOD NEWS ABOUT CHEMOTHERAPY

There's a range of possible side effects from chemotherapy: nausea, vomiting, hair loss, constipation or mouth ulcers. Chemotherapy can also, for example, affect your heart and lower your blood counts. Sexual problems are usually transitory, unlike surgery where the effects can be permanent. For details on how to cope with these issues, please read the following chapter, bearing in mind you may experience few or none of these.

Chemotherapy may reduce sperm production, affect potency, reduce your chance of pregnancy. Speak to your doctor about storing your sperm or eggs prior to treatment if you are concerned about your fertility. Pregnancy may not be possible unless by artificial means. There are unknown long-term risks to progeny (such as increased rate of tumors).

Treatment can also affect the way you feel about yourself. You may feel less attractive, for example, if your hair was your crowning glory and you lose it.

The effects of treatment for your breast, prostate and cervical cancer may make you feel that you are less desirable and cause you extreme distress. A frank and open expression of feelings, including lots of touching, stroking, kissing and cuddling, will go a long way to re-establishing intimacy with your partner.

The good news about chemotherapy

Chemotherapy can be used to cure certain cancers and, where a cure is not possible, can help you to live longer – and with fewer symptoms. Most childhood cancers, some aggressive lymphomas, Wilms' tumor and Ewing's sarcoma, to name but a few, can be cured successfully by chemotherapy.

In the case of adult cancers, the success rate of chemotherapy depends on a number of factors: the type of cancer, your age, your fitness, how far your cancer has progressed, where it has spread, your attitude and determination to pull through – the list goes on.

For many people, chemotherapy dramatically improves the quality of their lives by alleviating their painful and distressing symptoms – and by prolonging their lives. *One in four people who receive chemotherapy require no further treatment.* Many more achieve long-lasting remissions. In the light of this optimistic outlook, you may find it easier to put up with the short-term side effects, unpleasant as they can sometimes be.

... and the good news about side effects

- They do not last long.
- Relief is available for many of these effects, most of which disappear soon after treatment is stopped.
- Not everyone reacts in the same way.

Remember, the treatment you receive applies to you and no one else. Some people never lose their hair, others never get nausea, still others never vomit. It all depends on the type of drug you are given and for how long it is used.

- Your expectations can affect the way you react to chemotherapy. Some people get nauseous even before their treatment has started; conversely, you can improve your chance of avoiding or reducing side effects if you adopt a positive attitude.
- You can relieve some of your symptoms if you adjust your diet.

How chemotherapy is given

Chemotherapy agents are usually clear and colourless liquids, given by the hour, daily or even weekly. Some are administered by intravenous injection into a drip over several hours, or by a single injection under the skin, or into a muscle at varying intervals. Others may be given to you by mouth (pills, capsules, liquids), applied to your skin, or introduced via a catheter (a thin tube) into a specific area.

It can be given to you in hospital, a day centre, in your doctor's office, at home – it all depends on your particular treatment. In most instances, your doctor is likely to administer it in hospital so he can check on its effect and make any necessary adjustments to dosage.

Precautions you should take

Because of the nature of some chemotherapy drugs, you must tell your doctor if

- you are taking any other prescription or non-prescription medicine, including pain-relievers, laxatives, vitamins;
- you are allergic to any medicine – prescription or non-prescription;
- you are pregnant or intend to have children;
- you are breast-feeding an infant; or
- you have any other medical problems – no matter how minor they may seem to you. For example, tell your doctor if you have recently had (or been exposed to) an infection of any sort, in particular chickenpox, herpes zoster (shingles), or if you have any other condition such as kidney or liver disease.

Examples of life-saving chemotherapy agents[5]

It would be impossible in a book of this nature to list all the various drugs and the combinations in which they are given. Here is a short list (up-to-date as at May 1998) of some of the more well-known and potentially life-saving chemotherapy treatments from which your cancer specialist may choose.

Adriamycin/doxorubicin

A red-coloured solution, adriamycin is made from antibiotics. It is used successfully on its own or in combination with other chemotherapy drugs in the treatment of a range of cancers.

It is very effective, often offering long-term survival, in the treatment of acute leukemia, breast, Hodgkin's, lung, non-Hodgkin's lymphoma, ovary, neuroblastoma, sarcomas (soft-tissue cancers), and Wilms' tumor. It evokes *some* response in the treatment of many other cancers too numerous to mention. Adriamycin is administered intravenously.

Cisplatin

Cisplatin is a clear, colourless liquid that is used on its own or in combination with other chemotherapy drugs to alleviate the symptoms of tumors in the following organs: bladder, carcinoma of head and neck, lung, ovary, prostate, testicle, uterine cervix.

A combination of cisplatin and adriamycin occasionally achieves an excellent response in treating mesothelioma, a rare form of lung cancer linked to asbestos and usually difficult to treat. Cisplatin, when used in combination with other chemotherapy drugs to treat small ovarian cancers, achieves a 70-80 per cent success rate.[6]

Cisplatin is usually given over several hours via a slow, intravenous injection.

Cyclophosphamide (cytoxan/cycloblastin)

A clear, colourless solution, cyclophosphamide is unusual in that, in itself, it is not a cancer-killing drug, but becomes active when converted in the liver.

Cyclophosphamide can be used on its own or in combination with other chemotherapy drugs.

Cancers that usually respond to chemotherapy respond to cyclophosphamide. It is used to treat malignant lymphomas, multiple myeloma, acute and chronic leukemias, skin cancers such as mycosis fungiodes, and Kaposi's sarcoma. Solid tumors, cancer of the breast, ovary and uterine cervix, small-cell lung cancer, prostate cancer, and sarcomas all respond to cyclophosphamide. It is effective in the treatment of breast cancer which has spread to other parts of the body, and used in the treatment of pediatric cancers such as Ewing's sarcoma, neuroblastoma and rhabdomyosarcoma.

Cyclophosphamide is administered intravenously.

Fluorouracil (5-fu, adrucil)

Fluorouracil (flure-oh-YOOR-a-sill) rapidly enters every tissue in the body. Its action is so extensive, it is used to treat the symptoms of a range of malignant tumors, especially those of the bladder, breast, colon, pancreas (islet cell carcinomas), ovary, pancreas, prostate, skin, stomach, and cervix.

Fluorouracil is given as an intravenous injection or, in the case of skin cancers, as a cream. It can also be injected directly into an affected organ such as the liver when, for example, a bowel tumor has spread into it.

Methotrexate (mtx)

Depending on the type of cancer to be treated, methotrexate is an intravenous agent that can be used on its own or in combination with other agents.

On its own, it is used to treat breast cancer, and certain vaginal and uterine cancers associated with pregnancy – choriocarcinoma and hydatiform mole. In combination with other drugs, it is used to control acute leukemias, Burkit's lymphoma, breast, head and neck cancers, lympho-sarcoma, and secondary cancer that has spread to the lining of the brain. It is also used, in conjunction with surgery and radiation, to treat osteogenic sarcoma.

Good results are often achieved with methotrexate when it is given as additional therapy in the treatment of breast cancer following radical mastectomy.

Mitoxantrone (novantrone)

Similar, but not identical, to the way in which adriamycin works, mitoxantrone can successfully be used on its own as a first-line treatment for locally advanced breast cancer, or when it has spread to the lungs, lymph nodes, liver, bone and skin.

Recurrent or difficult-to-treat cases of non-Hodgkin's lymphoma have responded well to it. When administered in conjunction with another chemotherapy drug, cytarabine, mitoxantrone is effective in the treatment of adult acute lymphocytic leukemia (ALL) and chronic myelogenous leukemia. Mitoxantrone is given intravenously.

Radiotherapy

Radiotherapy is the use of radiation, X-rays or gamma rays, to destroy specific tumors, particularly in relatively confined areas. Radiotherapy is more specific than chemotherapy and is generally used to treat cancers that have not spread.

If you studied science at school, you may recall that all matter is made up of atoms, consisting of a central core, a nucleus, with electron particles revolving around it. Radiation appears to work by destroying the electrons. This, in turn, creates ions or charged particles which destroy the normal structure and function of molecules and, as with chemotherapy, prevents the cancer cells from dividing.

Rapidly dividing or malignant cells are more sensitive to radiation than cells that are at rest, so the decision to use radiotherapy is based on the cancer cells to be treated having a higher degree of sensitivity than the surrounding normal tissue.

As with chemotherapy and surgery, even if radiotherapy cannot treat your cancer it can be used most effectively to shrink it, which will relieve pain or bleeding, and to prevent the cancer from spreading. If your tumor is difficult to reach, your doctor may suggest radiotherapy to shrink it so it can be removed later, more easily, by surgery.

Since the 1970s, the success rate of radiotherapy has improved dramatically due largely to better and safer equipment. Some machines are now so accurate they can direct a beam at a tumor at any given depth without damaging the surrounding tissue.

How radiotherapy is given

Radiotherapy is administered through the skin by a beam aimed at the cancer, and takes as little as one to five minutes to deliver the required dose.

It can also be given by implanting tiny radioactive 'seeds' or needles (brachytherapy) near or into the tumor. This method is used most frequently to treat cancers of the oral cavity, oropharynx, cervix, and prostate. Implants have the advantage that they do not affect surrounding tissue. Most implants are left in place from one to six days, but in prostate cancer, for example, an implant may be left in permanently.

Another method is to inject radioactive ions bound to chemicals which concentrate in a specific tissue. Radioactive iodine, for example, injected into the bloodstream, will go directly to and destroy cancerous thyroid tissue without affecting any other parts of the body.

As with chemotherapy, the number, duration and frequency of radiotherapy treatments depends on several factors, including the type of cancer, where it is located and the stage to which it has progressed. Based on these, treatment can vary from a single dose to treatment five times a week for several weeks. The program can be intimidating if you're unprepared.

The area of your body to be treated is usually marked with gentian violet, and should not be washed off or else you will have to be re-painted. The vital areas surrounding the cancer may be protected by lead shields to prevent radiation injury to other parts of your body during the actual treatment. If you have ever undergone an X-ray or CT-scan, you will find the procedure familiar: you will be asked to lie completely still as the tube, or head, of the machine is positioned over the area to be treated. You will then be left alone for a few minutes, the whir of the machine your only indication that you are being treated.

During this time, your doctor and the technicians will communicate with you via a two-way intercom as they watch you on a monitor.

THE NOT-SO-GOOD NEWS ABOUT RADIOTHERAPY
- Radiotherapy, like chemotherapy, poses a serious risk to an unborn child, and so pregnancy is not advisable.
- Radiotherapy to certain parts of the body can cause problems. For instance, radiotherapy applied to the mouth area can cause teeth to decay; applied to the pelvic area, it can cause menopause-like symptoms and, in some cases, infertility for men and women. It is common practice for men and women to have their sperm or eggs stored in a sperm or egg bank prior to chemotherapy or radiotherapy so artificial insemination is possible at some later stage.
- Hair growth following radiotherapy may be patchy or thin; over time it should return to normal.
- Your skin can become extremely sensitive. For a time after treatment, some people claim they feel 'hot' where they were

treated. You can help ease the symptoms of radiotherapy by staying out of the sun, wearing sunblock or a hat, wearing soft clothing – and not rubbing or scratching treated skin.

Ask your doctor or nurse to advise you on what soaps, creams, deodorants and powders you can use, as many of them leave a coating on your skin that can interfere with treatment. Also, don't shave with a razor. If you have to shave, use an electric razor – but again, ask your doctor or nurse if it's OK to do so.

☞ There may be a reduction in your blood counts if large parts of your body are treated. If this is severe, it can always be corrected by a blood transfusion.

☞ Some people complain of fatigue and lack of energy, tiredness and need lots of rest. This is a normal response, but it may take time for you to get back your old drive.

☞ Some people have nausea and loss of appetite, or as a consequence of abdominal treatment, diarrhoea.

☞ Some people suffer no side effects at all. Expectations can affect the outcome. If you *expect* to suffer nausea and fatigue, you are more likely to do so.

THE REAL GOOD NEWS ABOUT RADIOTHERAPY

☞ Radiotherapy does not hurt; like X-rays, you cannot see or feel the rays.

☞ It will not leave you 'radioactive' – you will not glow in the dark!

☞ Radiotherapy can be used to treat areas that cannot be reached with surgery.

☞ There are fewer physical changes than with surgery (e.g. removal of breast or limb) or chemotherapy (loss of hair). Radiotherapy does not cause your hair to fall out unless treatment is aimed at your head.

☞ The chances of being free of the disease five years after treatment is 70-90 per cent in the case of early-stage non-Hodgkin's lymphoma, Hodgkin's disease, prostate cancer and early stage breast cancer.[7]

Hormone (endocrine) therapy

To understand how hormone therapy works, it is important to understand what a hormone is, and what it does.

Every function in your body is controlled by two major control systems which often interact with each other: the nervous system and the hormonal, or endocrine, system.

Hormones are chemical substances that travel to all parts of the body to regulate the function or growth of other cells, and are produced in the eight major endocrine glands: the pituitary, thyroid, parathyroid, adrenal, pineal, gonads, paraganglia and pancreas. All the cells in our body depend on hormones for their growth. In general, the hormonal system controls the chemical reactions inside and between cells (known as *metabolism*), the rate at which certain substances flow from cell to cell, and the growth of cells.

Hormone therapy can be administered by tablets or by injection. Treatment may last from only a few weeks, or indefinitely as with Tamoxifen, a widely used hormone agent used to treat certain kinds of breast cancer.

How hormone therapy works

Certain tumors depend to some extent on hormones for their growth. The purpose of hormone therapy is to prevent cell division by manipulating these hormones and so prevent tumors from growing.

Hormone therapies do not kill cancer cells, so they do not offer a cure. However, hormone therapy is highly effective in controlling symptoms and delaying the progress of advanced or widespread cancers. Prostate and breast cancer, in particular, react favourably to hormone treatment used in conjunction with chemotherapy or radiotherapy. Most hormones are given as adjuvant treatment to delay or prevent recurrence.

Sex hormones

The hormones we are concerned with are the sex hormones, estrogen and progesterone, which are secreted in women mainly by the ovaries and the adrenal glands (which lie above the kidneys). Estrogen promotes the growth and spread of all cells that define and maintain female sexual characteristics, while the primary function of progesterone is to prepare the womb for pregnancy, the breasts for feeding.

In men, the main sex hormone is testosterone, produced by the testes and the adrenals. There are various other male sex hormones which are less important than testosterone. Male sex hormones are referred to collectively as 'androgens'. Androgens are primarily involved in the development of male characteristics such as the sexual organs, skin thickness, muscle development, hair and bone growth – even enlarging the larynx to produce a deeper voice. They are used by weight lifters who want to develop bigger muscles.

Hormone therapy is aimed at blocking cell growth *in cancers that are hormone-sensitive*. As a rule, male hormones are used to treat cancers which occur in women; female hormones are used to treat cancers which occur in men. Breast cancer cells have estrogen receptors on them and so they will respond to a therapy that suppresses estrogen; prostate cancer cells have testosterone receptors on them and so they will respond to a therapy that suppresses testosterone. An example of a drug that does both is goserelin (Zoladex), which is used to treat advanced breast cancer in pre-menopausal women and prostate cancer in men.

Hormone therapy is a preferred method of treatment for breast cancer, as it adds more years to a patient's life than chemotherapy – with fewer or no side effects. It is also the main form of treatment in older men where surgery or radiotherapy can cause other problems.

SIDE EFFECTS OF HORMONE THERAPY

Hormone therapy can cause irregular periods in women, loss of potency in men. In both men and women it can cause hot flushes, affect sex drive, cause weight gain, make skin more sensitive to light. Growth of breast tissue in men is a common side effect of therapy with female hormones. In all cases, reducing the dose will almost always relieve these symptoms.

In the case of the agent Tamoxifen, clinical trials show that some women taking this hormone agent for breast cancer can develop uterine cancer. The benefits of Tamoxifen as a treatment for breast cancer are firmly established, far outweigh the potential risk of other cancers and, as in the case of Marcia (see Chapter 2), can even reverse cancer that has spread to other organs. If you are worried about the side effects of Tamoxifen, or any other drug for that matter, discuss your concerns with your doctor. Remember, the worst side effect you can experience is *that the treatment does not work.*

HORMONE THERAPY FOR BREAST CANCER

As I mentioned earlier, cancers grow at different rates and breast cancer is no exception, growing at different rates in different women. Also, a one-centimetre tumor contains about a billion cancer cells. This means that it could have been in your body *for many years before it became apparent.*

This, more than anything else, helps to explain why breast cancer is so difficult to treat, and why there is no need to rush into surgery overnight. Taking your time to recover from the shock of your diagnosis will give you the opportunity, when you are calmer, to discuss the best treatment option with your doctor.

Breast cancer affects men as well as women, although it is far less common among men.

HORMONE THERAPY FOR PROSTATE CANCER

Male hormones, especially testosterone, stimulate the growth of prostate cancer. To stop this process, female hormones may be given to decrease the amount of male hormones produced.

When prostate cancer produces severe symptoms or where it has recurred, hormone therapy may be used in conjunction with radiotherapy to relieve symptoms. The results are often dramatic: people who have been confined to bed because of bone pain can return to normal activities only a few days after receiving treatment. Surgery and radiotherapy are not viable options if prostate cancer has spread to other parts of the body. It also tends to occur in older men who may be unfit to withstand extensive surgery, so hormone therapy is the only viable alternative in such cases. In all cases, hormone therapy can result in remissions lasting several years. Most are given in pill form.

EXAMPLES OF HORMONE AGENTS FOR BREAST AND PROSTATE CANCER[8]

Aminoglutethimide (cytadren)
Aminoglutethimide blocks adrenal androgens in men, thus providing

an effective treatment for prostate cancer. It is also excellent in the treatment of breast cancer, as it blocks adrenal sex hormone production.

Treatment with aminoglutethimide can produce a skin rash but it goes away eventually.

Eulexin (flutamide)
Eulexin is another drug that targets androgens released by the adrenals which stimulate the growth of cancer in the prostate gland.

Eulexin is highly effective, but because it has no androgen effect on its own, it is used in conjunction with estrogen in the treatment of advanced prostate cancer where no previous treatment was given.

Fluoxymesterone (halotestin)
Fluoxymesterone is an effective hormone therapy used to treat advanced inoperable breast cancer in women who are *not* estrogen-sensitive.

Known as an androgenic hormone, Fluoxymesterone acts by stimulating the release of testosterone and so is a most effective anti-estrogen, also used if Tamoxifen fails to achieve the desired result.

Because androgens regulate bone growth, Fluoxymesterone cannot be used by people who have osteoporosis or are nursing mothers.

Goserelin acetate (zoladex)
An example of both an anti-estrogen and anti-testosterone, Goserelin is used to treat both locally extensive and widespread prostate cancer and advanced forms of breast cancer in pre-menopausal women.

Recent reports indicate that the use of goserelin and tamoxifen may prove even more effective in the treatment of advanced pre-menopausal advanced breast cancer. White or cream-coloured, goserelin is given as a subcutaneous injection into the abdomen.

Megestrol acetate (megace/megostat)
A synthetic, non-toxic hormone, megestrol acetate is an excellent treatment for recurrent, inoperable or widespread breast cancer.

Megestrol is a progesterone, although the reason for its anti-tumor activity is unclear. It is the least toxic therapy used in the treatment of breast cancer.

Tamoxifen (nolvadex)

Tamoxifen is an anti-estrogen pill used on its own or in combination with some chemotherapy drugs to treat advanced breast cancer in men and women who have passed menopause.

When tamoxifen is used as additional therapy for early-stage breast cancer, it prevents the recurrence of the original cancer, and prevents the development of new cancers in the other breast. At the time of writing (1998), tamoxifen is under trial for the *prevention* of breast cancer in healthy women. Recently, an FDA panel recommended the use of the osteoporosis drug, raloxifene. As with similar new drugs under trial – including idoxifene, droloxifene, toremifene, trioxifene, and zindoxifene – raloxifene is an estrogen *modulator*, so it may be a better long-term alternative than tamoxifen.

Immunotherapy and biological response modifiers

The basic function of the immune system is to identify anything that does not belong to our body so it can destroy it. How it does this is one of the miracles of life.

The immune system is made up of millions of different types of white blood cells. If bacteria, viruses or other micro-organisms enter the body, the white cells recognise them as foreign bodies and start multiplying aggressively in order to destroy them.

For example, as a result of you cutting yourself, bacteria penetrate your skin, start to grow and set up an infection. As soon as your immune system recognises these bacteria as foreign, white blood cells attack and destroy them. Pus is made of white blood cells that have been lost in the battle.

If the invader is a living thing such as bacteria, our immune system kills it; if the attacker is not alive – such as poison from a bee sting – it is eliminated.

The white cells making up our immune system are made up of *eosinophils*, which combat allergies and chronic parasitic infections, *neutrophils* (granulocytes), which fight bacterial infections, and *lymphocytes,* which attack viruses, transplanted cells and tumors. Lymphocytes are divided into two sub-groups: T-cells which are made in the thymus, and B-cells which are made in the bone marrow. B- and T-cells communicate with each other by way of the proteins they secrete, called *cytokines.*

White blood cells are not all located in the blood. They are distributed throughout the body, and some of them are strategically placed to defend against invasion. Called *macrophages*, they guard vital organs such as the lungs, liver, kidneys, as well as the central nervous system.

The word 'immune' comes from the Greek word for memory, the very attribute our immune system shares with our central nervous system. Having a good memory is essential to the smooth working of the immune system. The reason is simple: our bodies do not have a standing army of white cells large enough to deal with a major attack. To compensate for this, it keeps only a few copies of each type of white cell, but the moment these recognise a cell as foreign, the message goes out, 'Multiply!' The reaction time between the attack and a response can vary, and explains why, for example, there is a delay between the onset of flu and the routing of the virus by the immune system.

Our immune system can fail in three ways:

☞ It can overreact to a foreign substance as an *allergy*, perhaps the most common form of immune disorder.

☞ The immune system may fail to recognise a foreign substance and attack itself, causing an *auto-immune disease* such as rheumatoid arthritis or lupus.

☞ Cancer itself, or the treatments for it such as chemotherapy and radiotherapy, can damage the immune system's ability to fight infection, resulting in what is known as *immuno-deficiency*. In the case of AIDS (Acquired Immune Deficiency Syndrome), the invading virus simply overwhelms the immune system so it cannot defend itself against other infections.

How immunotherapy works

Immunotherapy, in the form of biological response modifiers, works by stimulating the immune system to attack cancer cells *as if they did not belong to our bodies*. In this unique way, they can, for example,

☞ hinder the growth of cancer cells;

☞ enhance the immune system's ability to fight them;

☞ make cancer cells more sensitive so our own immune system can destroy them;

☞ stimulate a cancer cell to become a normal cell;
☞ enable our bodies to repair normal cells damaged by, for example, chemotherapy or radiotherapy.

Although immunotherapy so far has been largely experimental, recent clinical successes indicate that it is already a potent way of treating certain cancers. What is most appealing about this type of treatment is that it can attack cancer that has spread to distant parts of the body. Moreover, the immune system targets only diseased cells and not healthy ones – unlike chemotherapy, immunotherapy does not attack ordinary dividing cells.

EXAMPLES OF BIOLOGICAL RESPONSE MODIFIERS

Interferons

Interferons are small proteins that are a normal part of the body's immune system. They promote T-cell response and hinder cell division, so they are extremely successful in treating hairy cell leukemia and chronic myelogenous leukemia.

Interferons have achieved significant success rates in the treatment of cutaneous T-cell lymphoma, low-grade lymphocytic leukemia, ovarian cancer and Kaposi's sarcoma. A 1995 report showed that patients with malignant melanoma treated with interferon and surgery showed a 20 per cent better survival rate than those treated with surgery alone.[9]

Some success has been achieved with interferons in treating gliomas, multiple myeloma, melanoma, and kidney cancer. Results in the treatment of bladder and intra-epithelial cervical cancer are encouraging. Current studies with Hodgkin's lymphoma and nasopharyngeal carcinoma are still being evaluated.[10]

Interleukins

Interleukins are hormone-like substances produced by lymphocytes in the immune system that cause other lymphocytes to grow and, in some instances, reverse immune deficiency. They are important in helping the immune system defend against infection and disease.

Interleukin-1 (IL-1) activates T-cells and stimulates bone marrow growth. Laboratory studies have shown that IL-1 has a direct anti-tumor effect on breast cancer and melanoma cells. Interleukin-2 (IL-2) has been remarkably successful in the treatment of widespread melanoma and is the first non-surgical therapy for kidney cancer approved in the USA.[11]

Colony-stimulating factors

Bone marrow, the source of all blood cells, is essential to the immune system. Colony-stimulating factors stimulate bone marrow cells to divide and differentiate into various white and red blood cells as well as platelets. Using CSFs to stimulate the production of white blood cells to fight infection *during chemotherapy*, doctors have been able to double, sometimes quadruple, successfully the dosages of chemotherapy to achieve even better results than they could before. The long-term outlook for the use of blood growth factors appears promising.

Monoclonal antibodies

Part of our natural defences against infectious agents are *antibodies* – proteins that seek out and help destroy invading micro-organisms known as *antigens*. For every type of antigen there is a matching antibody.

Monoclonal antibodies are made by injecting human cancer cells into mice so their immune systems make antibodies against these cells. The mouse cells that produce these antibodies are then removed and engineered to produce a hybrid cell, called a *hybridoma*. Hybridomas can be used to produce infinitely large quantities of pure monoclonal antibodies for use in humans. They are called monoclonal because they are made from one type of cell (*mono* means 'one').

Scientists have also found that when myeloma cells, which can be adapted to grow permanently in cell culture, are fused with anti-body-producing mammalian spleen cells, the resulting hybrid cells generate large amounts of monoclonal antibody.

Unlike other forms of therapy which attack all cells, monoclonal antibodies target only specific cells, so they produce few or no side effects. Also, monoclonal antibodies can be 'labelled' with radioactive iodine so they can be seen when they successfully locate, for example, colorectal tumor cells that have metastasised to other parts of the body.

Tumor necrosis factor

Whenever we have an infection, injury or inflammation, the macrophages in our body's immune system produces identical hormone-like substances called cachectin and tumor necrosis factor – TNF ('necrosis' comes from the Greek word 'to kill'). They are produced by specific white blood cells, and can be either beneficial or harmful.

At low levels they help to repair tissue damage and to fight germs; at high levels they are extremely toxic. In a remarkable feat of genetic engineering, scientists have been able to synthesise TNF to kill cancer cells. No one knows precisely how it does this, but it is believed it works by cutting off the developing blood supply in that area.

In a 1994 breakthrough at the Scripps Institute in La Jolla, California, scientists were able to shrink various solid tumors, including cancers of the lung, colon, breast and brain, by using TNF.[12] If successfully trialled in humans, synthesised TNF will offer a unique way of not only preventing cancer growth, but more especially, preventing metastasis.

Gene therapy

Cancer is the direct result of damaged genes, so the aim of gene therapy is to introduce genes into the body that will enable it to reverse or stop the cancer's lethal rampage.

This approach is revolutionary. Instead of giving you a drug to treat or control the symptoms of a genetic disorder, this therapy attempts to correct the basic problem by altering the genetic makeup of some of your cells. Gene therapy also represents a new way to increase the body's ability to recognise and shrink cancer cells. A normally quiescent gene that promotes cell growth is known as an oncogene – from the Greek word *ogkos* meaning 'mass' or 'tumor '(hence oncologist).

A 1995 report in the USA highlighted the promise of this approach.[13] Allovectin-7, the genetic material used to make a specific transplantation protein, was injected into the tumors of more than 40 patients; early results indicated the increased ability of the immune system to recognise the cells as cancer cells and to destroy them. They were effective against a number of different tumors, including melanoma, kidney and colon cancer.

Gene therapy has also been used in combination with stem cell treatment. Stem cells are the self-renewing 'mother' cells that give rise to all of the various types of blood cells. Since 1968, when the first bone marrow transplant between people who were not identical twins was successfully carried out, stem cells have been harvested from bone marrow and used to treat patients with otherwise incurable diseases. More recently, it was found that stem cells harvested from circulating blood (known as peripheral blood stem cells or PBS), for reasons still unknown, result in a more rapid recovery of certain key blood cells following transplantation than cells drawn from the marrow. In another new development, researchers successfully made PBS cells resistant to the toxic effects of chemotherapy by transferring resistance genes into them. In future, this means patients with advanced cancers will be able to undergo more intensive treatment without causing the damage to bone marrow that usually occurs during such treatment.

Gene therapy may also prove to be useful in treating pre-cancerous conditions, especially where people have a genetic predisposition to certain cancers, for example, familial adenomatous polyposis. This is a condition in which polyps develop in the colon, and, unless surgically removed, usually progress to cancer. Scientists found that by interbreeding mice with intestinal polyps with mice with a genetically-induced shortage of an enzyme called DNA methyltransferase, they were able to reduce the number of polyps by 60 per cent. When the methyltransferase levels were reduced even further using a drug known as 5-aza-dC, the number of polyps fell by 98 per cent.[14]

Other treatment options

New treatments are constantly being developed. Some are variations on (or extensions of) existing therapies – new drugs for use in chemotherapy, for example; others are completely novel. Some are still under trial, others are gaining acceptance as their success rates grow, still others have yet to make it to trial stage. Drugs commonly used to treat certain cancers are often subsequently found to be helpful in treating others. There are so many new treatments, it would be impossible to list them all, so I have a selected a few as examples.

RECENTLY INTRODUCED DRUGS
Gemcitabine (2', 2'-difluorodeoxycytidine)

The symptoms of pancreatic cancer do not usually appear until the disease is well advanced, making this type of cancer one of the most difficult to treat. It is rarely curable.

Preliminary studies of a new drug, Gemcitabine, have shown promising results with patients who are no longer candidates for surgery or who are resistant to other chemotherapy drugs.

The Food and Drug Administration in the USA approved the use of this new drug in early 1995.

Navelbine-r (vinorelbine tartrate)

Vinorelbine is a semi-synthetic plant alkaloid which was initially developed in France in the 1980s. After extensive trials, Navelbine was approved by the FDA for treatment of squamous-cell carcinoma, adenocarcinoma and advanced non-small-cell lung cancer in people who cannot undergo surgery because of the extent of their disease. Navelbine is less toxic than previous drugs.

Taxol

Taxol is an exciting new drug made from yew trees that is being used successfully to treat ovarian cancer, from which over 20 000 women die each year in the USA. Current trials throughout the world show that Taxol holds even greater promise for the treatment of breast and lung cancer, possibly many other cancers.

Camptothecin (cpt-11)

An example of an exciting new group of drugs – topoisomerase inhibitors – CPT-11 works by preventing cancer cells dividing endlessly. Administered intravenously, it is currently used for the treatment of melanomas and solid tumors, in particular, pre-treated breast cancer that has spread elsewhere.

Several studies show that CPT-11 has anti-tumor activity in adenocarcinomas of the colon and non-small-cell lung cancer, as well as cervical and ovarian cancer. Complete remissions have been achieved with CPT-11 where several other chemotherapy drugs failed to achieve any response.

Isotretinoin (13-cis-retinoic acid)

A drug often used to treat severe acne may offer new hope for young children with a rare and deadly form of childhood leukemia, juvenile chronic myelogenous leukemia.

In a pilot study in 1994 of the drug, which is a derivative of vitamin A, all the children had lengthy remissions, making them better candidates for bone marrow transplants – the most effective long-term and curative therapy for this rare disease.[15]

Capcitabine (xeloda)

This treatment received accelerated approval by the FDA in April 1998 for patients with metastatic breast cancer resistant to other drugs. Xeloda, taken orally, is converted by the body to 5-fluorouracil (see page 128).

Letrozole (femara)

Letrozole is a promising new estrogen blocker for advanced breast cancer in post-menopausal patients whose cancer resists other anti-estrogens. It is still under trial.

PHOTO-DYNAMIC THERAPY (PDT)

In PDT therapy, a light-sensitive drug known as HPD (hemato-porphyrin-derivative) is injected into the body and is absorbed by the cancer. An endoscope is then used to shine a laser light onto it, producing a chemical reaction which kills the tumor cells. Surrounding tissue is unaffected.

It has shown remarkable results – in many cases, complete remission – in the treatment of early bladder cancer, early esophageal and gastric cancers, basal cell carcinoma, Kaposi's sarcoma, and early lung cancer. PDT is effective in the treatment of certain recurrent breast cancers of the chest, cervix, vagina and vulva, cancers of the larynx, mouth, head and neck tumors and non-melanoma skin cancers.[16]

Approved for use by the FDA in the USA, PDT is also used in the Netherlands and Japan, and in Australia for certain brain tumors.

LIPOSOMES

Although not a treatment in themselves, liposomes provide an unusual link between the various treatments.

The dream of scientists since the turn of the century has been to target specific cells without affecting surrounding ones. This is now possible thanks to the use of liposomes, more popularly known for their use in cosmetics.

As you know, oil and water don't mix. Liposomes are minute hollow spheres made of a lipid (fatty) membrane on the outside, an aqueous solution inside. In a remarkable feat of chemistry, liposome molecules can be made to encapsulate liquid cancer drugs to target specific cancers, for example, brain cancers. The brain is protected by a barrier that keeps out anything that can upset it. Until recently, the only way a drug could be used to attack a brain tumor was to drill holes into the head of the patient. This works in treating surface tumors but does not reach deeper cancers.

By encapsulating daunorubicin inside liposomes and then attaching these liposomes to molecules of a protein called transferrin that can pass through the brain barrier, doctors can ensure that this powerful anti-cancer drug is absorbed into the brain.

Following an intensive trial which started in 1991 in the USA on moderate to severe AIDS-related Kaposi's sarcoma patients, the FDA approved the use of encapsulated doxorubicin in 1995 for the treatment of Kaposi's sarcoma. The trial, which is ongoing, showed that the long-term use of DOX-SL (stealth liposomal doxorubicin HCl) is highly effective, and with almost no side effects.[17]

At the time of writing, clinical trials with liposome-encapsulated doxorubicin are being carried out at the Cancer Center of the University of Pennsylvania by Dr Joseph Treat to study the effects of this therapy in several types of solid tumors, including breast, lung, ovarian, prostate, small-cell lung cancer and leukemia.

Other trials on solid tumors have shown that liposomal vincristine (another powerful anti-cancer drug) is ready for a further round of trials.[18]

Using encapsulated drugs means far higher doses of drugs can be given, with minimal or no side effects.

It seems highly likely that liposomes may be used in the future to correct defective or missing genes.[19]

Clinical trials

Before you can be given any treatment to cure your cancer, control your pain, or reduce the side effects, it has to be tested. Tests conducted in a test tube or a laboratory environment with animals are referred to as *in vitro*. If these tests are promising, they are then considered for testing *in vivo*, that is, in a living body. Medicine tends to be conservative, so it can take many years before a treatment is deemed effective or safe enough to be used.

Testing new drugs is also expensive. A single drug takes, on average, US$86m and nine years to go from the first test to final approval. The cost to drug manufacturers is multiplied when you consider that of the 10 000 new substances tested annually in the USA, only about eight make it to the clinical trial stage, and of these, for every five that start out, only one is successful.

A clinical trial is an organised study usually conducted with people who have a life-threatening disease, and designed to:

(a)   test a new treatment; or

(b)   test new ways of using known treatments; or

(c)   compare known treatments against new ones.

There are many hundreds of treatments currently under trial. For example, in April 1997, 100 gene therapy trials were awaiting approval by the US government.[20] Many people who could benefit from clinical trials are never given the chance to take part in them, and you might only be offered the chance to take part if your doctor or hospital is participating in a trial. Alternatively, there are many drugs and treatments under clinical trial that are available on a 'compassionate use', case-by-case basis where standard treatment is ineffective, no response to conventional treatment has been achieved, or the cancer has recurred. Ask your doctor about them.

If your doctor does offer you the chance to take part in a trial, find out as much about it as you can beforehand, obtain a copy of the plan known as the *protocol* from one of the doctors conducting the study. Be aware that trials for cancer treatments usually take place in three phases.

PHASE 1

A Phase 1 trial is aimed at finding out the best way to give a new treatment and how much of it can safely be given. It is usually easier for you to get into a Phase 1 trial, since it is nothing more than a study to find the optimum dose.

There are risks attached to this phase, even though the treatment has been well tested in the laboratory and in animals. Because of this, treatment in Phase 1 is only given to a small number of people with extremely advanced cancer who are considered to have little or no chance of recovery with conventional therapy.

PHASE 2
A Phase 2 trial is designed solely to test whether the treatment can produce measurable results on one type of cancer. Again, it is only on patients with advanced cancer that participate. For example, patients with breast cancer who have become resistant to standard treatment may be treated in a Phase 2 trial.

Patients are considered to have achieved a *response* if a tumor shrinks by at least a 50 per cent and stays like that for at least a month, a *partial response* if some tumor remains, a *complete response* if no detectable tumor remains. Response times vary from person to person: some treatments create more lasting responses than others.

Phase 2 trials are conducted on larger numbers of people, usually groups of 20 to 50 patients, so any side effects produced can be more easily measured.

PHASE 3
Phase 3 trials are aimed at comparing two treatments for a particular type of cancer in order to determine which one is better This usually means comparing the current preferred treatment against one that achieved good results in Phase 2.

The key objective in Phase 3 is to determine if the new treatment results in better survival, but quality of life and side effects are also measured. Some Phase 3 trials can involve thousands of people.

Phase 3 trials are 'randomised': patients are given one treatment or the other, but who gets what is random. The group that receives the standard treatment is known as the 'control group'. The only time a 'control group' is given no treatment is if no treatment is the standard form of treatment.

A 'double-blind' study is one in which patients – even their doctors – do not know which of two treatments they are receiving. In studies such as this, one group may receive standard treatment while the other receives the drug under trial; one group may receive a placebo (an inert substance), the other receives the drug under trial.

I cannot urge you strongly enough to make every effort to find out what is available to make absolutely sure that the treatment being offered to you has not been overtaken by some new discovery. Taking this approach saved my life; it could save yours.

eight

side effects of cancer and its treatments

◠

'Your pain is the breaking of the shell
that encloses your understanding.'

KAHLIL GIBRAN

There is a downside to almost all medical treatments; those used for cancer are no exception. The difficult nature of the disease means that the treatment often has to be harsh to be effective, often causing side effects to some degree or other. Generally speaking, the effects of not treating cancer are far worse than any of the potential side effects of the treatments for it.

Discuss the likely side effects of your treatment with your doctor if you are anxious about how you will respond. Bear in mind that some treatments produce no side effects, and that even if they do, not everyone responds in the same way; if someone you know did not tolerate a treatment well, this does not mean you will do likewise. Further, most side effects – losing your hair, for example – are usually temporary, and many can be controlled; drugs, like granisetron (Kytril) and ondansetron (Zofran), have all but eliminated the nausea and vomiting that can occur with chemotherapy or radiotherapy. Similarly, there is almost always something your doctor can do to relieve symptoms like fatigue, bleeding, infection, pressure sores, agitation and confusion. Contrary to what most people believe or expect, pain is not the most common side effect of cancer or its treatments, but it is probably the most treatable.

The importance of diet during treatment

Changing your diet won't reverse the course of your cancer, but it can make an appreciable difference to the way you respond to treatment.

Some treatments, by their very nature, damage cells which need all the support they can get in order to repair themselves. In some cases, altering your diet may even be life-saving if, for example, your sense of taste or smell has been affected so you are put off certain foods or simply don't feel like eating at all.

Many alternative diets recommend reducing, even eliminating, the intake of proteins. This can be dangerous: if you lose more than 30-50 per cent of your body protein stores, you can die.[21]

In general, you should attempt to prevent any deficiency in your nutritional intake by maintaining a balanced diet based on the four major food groups: fruit and vegetables; fish, meat and poultry; cereals and breads; dairy products.

Additional vitamins and minerals are only beneficial if you are unable to maintain a balanced diet. Commercial liquid food supplements can provide you with all the essential vitamins and minerals your body needs, should you find that eating solid foods causes problems.

Speak to your doctor or dietician if your treatment affects you in any way. Cancer councils in all countries also have excellent booklets with useful hints to help you through your treatment program.

Here is a short list of some side effects of treatments – and the ways in which you can deal with them, based on my own experiences and those described in *The Manual of Clinical Oncology* (3rd edition, 1996), and booklets issued by the National Cancer Institute in the USA and the Anti-Cancer Council of Victoria, Australia.

Loss of appetite (anorexia) and difficulty in eating

In most societies, a good appetite is seen as a sign of health and sociability, and vice versa. Cancer, and the treatments for it, can often cause you to lose your appetite or make eating difficult. For example, cancer of the pancreas, ovaries and the outer lining of the bowel can cause feelings of fullness, nausea, vomiting and cramp. This feeling of fullness can also be caused by a tumor in the stomach, or by an enlarged internal organ pressing on it. This is a feeling I know well. I looked as if I were nine months pregnant when my spleen swelled to 28 centimetres in length and pressed hard against most of my internal organs. It made me feel so bloated that I could hardly eat. The only way I could sustain myself was by sipping thirteen glasses of fruit, vegetable and raw liver juices a day.

Eating properly during treatment is essential to maintain your energy, help damaged cells repair themselves, reduce your risk of infections, and help prevent side effects. Drinking is just as important, as cells destroyed by chemotherapy or radiotherapy release, amongst other things, a substance called uric acid, which is filtered by the kidneys and passed out of the body through urine. It is essential that you drink large amounts of water to flush out these potentially harmful chemicals.

No one really knows what causes anorexia (lack or loss of appetite) in people with cancer, and attempts to remedy it are not very effective unless the cancer growth itself can be controlled. Steroids can help you get back an appetite, but they also suppress your body's immune system, cause or aggravate diabetes and gastritis, and increase the breakdown of muscle.

Here are some guidelines to help you overcome some of the problems you may face:

- Eat your favourite foods and keep delicious snacks at hand.
- Eat smaller meals or snacks instead of three regular meals.
- Walk before meals to stimulate your appetite.
- Drink weak tea, soda water, jelly to increase liquid intake.
- Enjoy an alcoholic beverage with your food (check with your doctor first).
- Change your mealtime routine: light candles, put on soft music, dress for dinner, eat out with friends.
- Experiment with new foods and recipes.
- Get 'Meals on Wheels' or pre-cooked meals if you live alone or can't be bothered cooking.
- Avoid greasy foods.

If your food still doesn't taste right despite all these hints, try the following:

- In preference to red meat, reduce the urea content of your diet by eating white meats, eggs and dairy products including ice cream.
- Marinate red meats in soy sauce, fruit juice or wine: cook with stronger seasoning.
- Eat your food cold or at room temperature.
- Eat foods that are tart: pickles, vinegar, lemonade frozen in ice trays.

Difficult in swallowing (dysphagia)

Difficulty in swallowing can be caused by a number of problems, including a tumor in the chest or stomach, or as a result of large doses of steroids and antibiotics giving rise to *candida* or thrush: tiny blisters on the tongue and down the food-pipe. Nystatin and other anti-bacterials are routinely given before and during treatment to overcome this often-painful condition.

Intravenous chemotherapy and radiation treatment to the face area can cause vitamin deficiency and make swallowing difficult as a result of a sore or dry mouth. You can alleviate these symptoms by trying any one or all of the following hints:

- Avoid foods that cause you pain.
- Fix any dental problems before you start treatment.
- Brush your teeth regularly with a soft brush.
- Rinse your toothbrush well after use and store it in a dry place.
- Use anti-bacterial powders and mouthwashes.
- Avoid mouthwashes with large amounts of salt or alcohol.
- Suck ice cubes, mints, sweets.
- Rinse your mouth frequently with baking soda mixed with water.
- Avoid tobacco and alcohol.
- Apply mild lip balm jelly to your lips. Some people say chafed lips are best treated with 'bag balm' (used for cow udders) which is obtainable from veterinary stores.

If excessive salivary production becomes uncomfortable or makes swallowing painful, tell your doctor. There are ways to treat this problem.

Difficulty in breathing (dyspnea)

This is perhaps the most distressing symptom of cancer. It can occur as a result of a tumor in the neck or lungs, a build-up of fluid in the abdominal area, congestion of the lymphatic system, a reduction in the number of oxygen-carrying red blood cells. It's enough to make anyone panic.

At one point in my first bout with cancer, my red blood cell count had dropped so low and its oxygen-carrying capacity was so severely diminished, that I experienced the most distressing symptoms: palpitations, dizziness, extreme exhaustion, shivering, and breathlessness. I was forever trying to suck in air without relief. At one stage, it took me ten minutes to catch my breath for every two steps I took. Turning over in bed was like running a marathon. I was lucky: these symptoms were relieved whenever I had a blood transfusion.

Loss of hair (alopecia)

You can lose the hair on your head and other parts of your body as a result of radiotherapy and chemotherapy. This usually starts two to three weeks after treatment begins, but the hair invariably grows back after treatment stops. Your hair may grow back while you're still having treatment; it may not grow back in the same color or texture as before. Hair loss is usually preceded by an itching or painful scalp.

Many people choose from a variety of wigs to cover up hair loss, often daring to try out new colours, new styles. Women have an easier time with a wide choice of colourful scarves, turbans, berets and hats – headgear that would draw unwelcome attention to a man.

- Use a sunscreen, sunblock, hat or scarf to avoid exposure to the sun.
- Use a soft bristle brush and a mild shampoo.
- Use low heat when drying your hair.
- Don't perm your hair, get a semi-permanent dye, or use brush rollers to set your hair.
- Sew towelling inside your wig to prevent irritation and absorb perspiration.
- Buy satin pillow cases – they're are easier to clean than cotton ones.
- Use a portable vacuum cleaner to clean your sheets, especially before washing them. Better still, wear a scarf or turban to bed.

Nausea and vomiting

Chemotherapy and radiotherapy can cause nausea and vomiting, but, as I stated earlier, this can vary from person to person, from treatment to treatment. Some people never vomit or feel nauseous, others feel slightly nauseated, still others can be severely nauseated for a short time during or after a treatment. These symptoms can almost always be treated.

Your doctor has a wide range of drugs, known as *anti-emetics,* to help suppress or stop nausea and vomiting. In some cases, it may be necessary to use more than one drug to get relief. One combination or other is bound to work for you. You can also help yourself by following these useful tips:

- Avoid large meals; eat smaller ones throughout the day.
- Drink before or after meals, not with meals. Avoid fizzy drinks.
- Eat and drink slowly.
- Avoid sweet, fried, or fatty foods.
- Eat food cold or at room temperature to avoid strong smells.
- Eat dry foods (cereal, toast, crackers) before getting up if you are affected by nausea in the morning.
- Don't lie down for at least two hours after you've finished your meal.
- Avoid eating for a few hours before treatment if you get nauseous during treatment.
- Suck ice cubes, mints, or sour sweets – but not if you have mouth or throat sores.
- Avoid smells that bother you: cooking, smoke, perfume.
- Prepare and freeze meals in advance for when you don't feel like cooking.
- Don't wear tight-fitting clothes.
- Breathe deeply and slowly if you feel nauseated.
- Distract yourself by chatting with friends or family members, listening to music, or watching a movie or TV show.

Pain

How would you describe pain? A bad feeling, severe discomfort, distress, hurt, sore, lousy, despair, like nothing on earth, like slow death? No two people describe pain in exactly the same way for one good reason: pain is so internal, so personal it belongs to no one else but you. Dr Albert Schweitzer, a medical missionary, founder of the leper colony in Lambaréné in French Equatorial Africa, and winner of the Nobel Peace Prize in 1952, once described pain as 'a more terrible lord of mankind than death itself'.

You may wince at the prospect of pain, but you can usually bear it if you know it will be short-lived. However, it can make even the bravest of us shrink if we think it will last for some time, or that it cannot be relieved. Not even the soothing words or the gentle touch of the most sympathetic and compassionate person is likely to help if pain persists, becomes unrelenting, exhausting, demoralising.

I thought the worst pain possible for anyone to experience was when I felt the pulpy crunch of a needle sliding into my hip bone for my first bone marrow biopsy. It was, however, nothing compared to the pain I felt following surgery for my lung cancer. According to doctors, a lobectomy (removal of part or all of a lung) is the most agonising of all medical experiences. Two women I know well have had the same operation and tell me it's more painful than childbirth; both agreed with my description that it's like having the inside of your chest continually scraped with a broken bottle.

Pain that is unrelieved causes unnecessary suffering, prevents you from enjoying even the simplest pleasures of life, limits your choices, and devalues your sense of worth. Prolonged pain can also affect your appetite and sleep, so the resulting loss of nutrition and fatigue weakens you even further, leads to irritability and depression, and eventually affects your rate of recovery. Specialists call this unhappy state of affairs the 'terrible triad': suffering, sleeplessness and sadness. It is as hard on your family as it is on you. Pain can rob you of hope, especially if you feel that it is an indication of the progress of your disease. Chronic, unrelieved pain may even make you reject treatment that could otherwise save your life.

The whole experience is one of such desperate helplessness that some people say they would welcome death if only it meant an end to the pain. It's not unusual for people to contemplate suicide when their pain becomes unbearable, when they're depressed, and feel they've lost control over the situation. In most cases, any thoughts of suicide quickly vanish once they receive adequate pain relief. The interesting thing is that contrary to popular understanding, most cancers do not cause pain; those that do can usually be effectively managed.

WHY WE EXPERIENCE PAIN

Pain is not an automatic companion to cancer and even when it is involved, it is not always persistent, more often intermittent. Cancer pain can be caused by recent surgery, by a tumor pressing on a nerve, organ or vessel, by the blockage of a blood vessel or the urinary tract, or by an infection or swelling.

Pain acts as a warning signal that something is wrong. You must tell your doctor immediately if you have any pain, no matter how insignificant it may seem to you at the time. Unrelieved acute or severe pain can often cause a chain of cardiac and respiratory problems and other metabolic events which can threaten your life.[1]

Pain is a physical response, but it can be increased a hundred-fold the more anxious and fearful you get. Your doctor can provide you with physical relief and, to some extent, ease your emotional pain by reassuring you of a positive outcome. You can help reduce the intensity of your suffering by focusing on the gain rather than the pain – and by trying some of the techniques described below (see 'How to cope with pain').

PAIN CONTROL AND PREVENTION

There is a growing acknowledgement among doctors and other caregivers who work with cancer patients that pain prevention is not only more satisfactory from your point of view than pain relief, it has real medical benefits: less time in hospital, lower costs, a quicker return to normal life. If you are given relief only when your pain has reached monumental proportions, you may have to be given larger doses, 'rescue doses', in order to control it, and so suffer the added problems of feeling 'bombed out', giddy and nauseous.

But there are still some pockets of resistance to pain prevention. For example, your doctor expects the relief from the drug she has prescribed for you to last for four to six hours, so she does not mark your prescription 'As needed'. Your pain returns sooner, you want relief, but your nurse has no authority to give it to you. Instead of compassion, there is confrontation.

The argument put forward by some doctors and caregivers is that providing pain relief – particularly morphine – can turn you into a drug addict, despite a growing body of evidence that morphine taken solely to prevent pain is not only the most effective method available, it is also *not* addictive unless you have a history of psychological disturbance or substance abuse. Moreover, pain prevention requires lower doses of morphine, so mental dullness and other side effects can be avoided.[2] People in pain who receive morphine don't get high, they get relief. When addicts take morphine, their quality of life goes down; when non-addicts take it, their quality of life goes up. I have little doubt that the pro-euthanasia movement would lose most of its following if morphine, called 'God's own medicine' by William Osler, became the drug of first choice for cancer pain.

Pain does not always entail alleviation with morphine, nerve-blocks, nerve stimulation, surgery or radiotherapy. Depending on the situation and your sensitivity, non-steroid anti-inflammatories, tranquillisers, anti-histamines, cortisone, anti-depressants and acupuncture can be used. Ask what options can be made available to you – but forget about heroin. Contrary to what some people believe, studies in Britain in the 1980s have confirmed that heroin has *no* advantages over any other painkiller.[3]

Unless you demand it, pain control should not knock you senseless. You may be prepared to put up with a certain amount of pain as long as this enables you to maintain some control over, and add quality to, your life. If you're not prepared to put up with pain and are willing to be rendered semi- or fully comatose by a pain-killing drug, I believe that it is your right to demand it, and no one should refuse you. Good management of cancer pain involves continuous monitoring, assiduous assessment and providing you with round-the-clock dosages of *effective* painkillers. Those who care for you should ask you frequently about your pain and use *your* report as their guideline, not theirs. The World Health Organisation, most oncologists and various studies[4] agree that cancer pain is, in general, still unrelieved and under-medicated, and that round-the-clock administration with additional 'as needed' doses should be the guiding principle of pain relief.

There are undoubtedly many reasons why there is poor assessment of pain, especially in busy outpatient clinics. You may not report your pain because you think that it is a sign your disease is worse, that it will distract your doctor from treating the underlying problem, or because you are concerned about becoming tolerant of drugs or dislike their side effects; your doctor may not provide you with adequate relief because she is more concerned about possible side effects, including addiction, than possible benefits, including an improved quality of life. If your needs are not met, demand to go to a pain clinic. There is no reason why you should suffer pain. This is as true of children as it is of adults.

It is untrue that children do not suffer the same pain as adults. Children are either unable or unwilling to complain about pain either because they fear needles, view their pain as some form of punishment, or because their parents view pain as a sign of weakness. A 1988 report by the Australian National Health and Medical Research Council points out that, as with many adults, children tend to lie quietly and withdraw from those around them when their pain is severe.[5] If your child is seriously ill and cries, it is almost certain he or she is in pain and should be treated accordingly – and immediately.

Everyone has a different pain threshold; everyone handles pain-relief medicine differently. Your family may be concerned about you being over-medicated, or even deny that you are in pain in order to avoid facing the possibility that your disease is progressing. You all need to talk about it, candidly. Your family and other caregivers need to remind themselves that as it is your pain that needs treating, only *you* can know what is enough or not; only *you* know how much you can or cannot bear.

Some people may be in remission for 10 or 20 years but continue to have chronic pain from their treatment. They are 'cancer-free' but are still experiencing 'cancer-related pain'; they are often not believed about their pain or offered appropriate treatment for it.

Here are some guidelines for dealing with pain:

- Report any new pain promptly to your doctor.
- Describe the intensity of your pain on a scale of 1 to 10.
- Describe where the pain is and if there is anything that seems to make it worse.
- Take your medication as prescribed and report any side effects immediately.

☞ Remind yourself that your emotional state and the degree to which you are stressed can increase the severity of your pain.

☞ Remember that pain does not build character; people who believe in the credo 'No pain, no gain' or that 'Only real people go the distance' are not cancer patients.

How to cope with pain

Time flies when you're having fun, drags when you're in pain; minutes feel like hours, hours like days. The more intense the pain, the longer it seems to last, the greater your suffering. The type and strength of the analgesic you are given can also affect your sense of time. As a rule, the more pain relief you receive, the more your sense of time is altered. You may recall the last time you received a particularly strong medication, and how you seemed to lose track of time, how 'spaced out' you felt. As Dr Larry Dossey points out in his book, *Space, Time & Medicine*, pain can be lessened if you lose track of time – and there is nothing that can create a sense of timelessness more than meditation (see Chapter 12).[6]

You can also modify your sense of time and subdue brief episodes of pain by focusing on something or someone external: television, your favourite music, radio, reading, praying, talking. Many people use guided imagery to distract themselves from their pain. For example, some people focus on their cancer and imagine it being eaten by sharks, others concentrate on what they think their cancer looks like, and then picture their white cells shooting them; still others imagine they are playing chess or draughts and, with the white pieces as white cells, the black pieces as cancer cells, win every game.

You can expand your sense of time and distract yourself from your pain by engaging in exercise you can manage and, preferably, enjoy: tai chi, walking, bowls, tennis, yoga, fishing. I have found no activity that comes closer to matching the sense of timelessness of meditation than gardening. Setting aside a part of your day for these activities will also help you regain control over what you do, and help you adopt a more optimistic attitude towards your eventual recovery.

If your pain is so intense that you are confined to bed, you may need to deal with it at different levels: drugs for the physical pain, understanding for your emotional pain, counselling for your psychological and spiritual pain.

You can also use your body's own natural painkillers. Athletes talk about achieving a 'high' after breaking through the pain barrier when they compete. The reason for this is that the body produces large proteins in the brain called *endorphins*, meaning the 'morphines within', which suppress pain messages. The 'high' that athletes get is an excess of endorphins; they are, quite literally, 'high'. It stands to reason that you can overcome pain by stimulating the release of these naturally-occurring substances by doing anything that makes you feel good: helping others, laughing, making love, exercising, hoping, meditating.

Pain always seems worse when we have to deal with it alone. We seem to cope much better when there is contact and communication, either in a group or with another individual.

A NOTE FOR FAMILY AND FRIENDS

You can help to ease the pain of the one you love by getting them to discuss their fears and anxieties.

Offer them love, understanding, some expression of tenderness. Show them you care. Let them set the agenda. Talk about what they want to talk about, even if you think you could handle the pain better if you were in their position. Pain recedes in the face of love – surely stronger than any other endorphin-releasing stimulus.

Sexual side effects

Quality of life for most people includes maintaining intimate relationships and expressing themselves as sexual beings. Cancer and the side effects of treatment can affect your sex life, lower your self-esteem, make you feel less confident. Overcoming these problems requires an adjustment, a rearranging of priorities, and an open expression of these concerns between you and your doctor; even more, then, is it necessary between you and your partner. People who have lost intimacy in their lives are likely to feel that no one cares about them, so they lose hope, stop trying to fight on.

Your age, your previous sexual attitudes and practices, the type of cancer you have and the treatment you receive all need to be considered. What is normal for you may not be normal for someone else. Your idea of good sex and intimacy may be different from someone else's. You may believe older people automatically lose interest in sex when in fact most people never do. You may feel that once you've had cancer, you will never have sex again when in fact most people do.

Two particular fears people with cancer seem to have is that intercourse will stimulate the recurrence of their cancer, and that sex can be harmful. If you have these fears, put them aside. The only limitations are that intercourse should be avoided temporarily following pelvic surgery when it can strain an incision and cause bleeding, and that chemotherapy or radiotherapy may weaken your immune system which puts you at greater risk of contracting a sexually transmitted disease.

It is impossible in a book of this nature to cover every possible sexual side effect which might occur, and the issue of pregnancy and cancer is particularly complex. Ask your doctor to explain all possible side effects and other matters to you. If she is embarrassed or unable to answer your questions to your satisfaction, ask her to refer you to a psychiatrist, a counsellor or a sex therapist. The explanations below may answer some or all of your concerns, or provide you with a starting point for further discussions.

How your feelings can affect sexual function

Negative emotions can affect your sex life. Sadness, despondency and depression can all reduce your desires, especially if you are fatigued, lethargic, in pain, or affected by the drugs you take.

Your anxieties can also take their toll. Your image of yourself may be radically altered by what you see in the mirror, or what you think someone expects of you. Will my husband still find me desirable with only one breast? What will my wife say when I can't get or maintain an erection? What does my partner think about my incontinence? Will I be able to achieve orgasm? Will I still be able to have children?

You may have placed great store in your looks, regarded them as your best attribute, felt good only when you looked good. You may become ashamed, even resentful, of your body if it starts to change, and if you feel you no longer have any control over it. These feelings will remain largely unresolved as long as discussion about them is regarded as 'off limits' by you and your doctor, or you and your partner – and as long as you fail to recognise there is more to you than your mortal frame, more to you than your looks.

It is often difficult for people without cancer to appreciate how you feel at this time. This lack of empathy is hard to face, especially when people say, 'Don't you have more important things to consider?' Or, 'Is that all you can think about?' Such responses reflect a lack of understanding of the key role sex plays in many people's lives. There are few other events that can remind us more of our mortality than being deprived of the very act that symbolises life.

How women can overcome sexual side effects
Breast cancer
Your response to breast surgery will depend on the treatment you receive: surgery, chemotherapy, radiotherapy, hormone therapy. Your emotional responses are likely to include concerns about whether the cancer has been properly removed, if it has spread, if you still have a role to play as a woman, mother, wife, lover – or all four.

Surgery can produce feelings of numbness, discomfort, and tingling on the chest wall where the breast was. Contrary to popular belief, radical mastectomies are rarely performed as they resulted in gross disfigurement and impairment of shoulder and arm movement – and they did nothing to increase life span. Nowadays, women are more likely to have a total mastectomy with axillary node dissection which involves removing the nipple, breast tissue and lymph nodes in the armpit only. Numbness occurs in the back of the arm, but it is usually temporary, although in some women it can be permanent; some women speak of phantom nipple sensation experienced as itching or pain.

Segmental or partial mastectomy, or tyelectomy – commonly known as lumpectomy – is the removal of only the tumor and a healthy margin of breast tissue around it for safety's sake. This is sometimes followed by radiation therapy, which can cause scarring (in women with fair skin), itchiness, tenderness or changes in breast size and shape.

Some chemotherapy and hormone treatments can interfere with the production of sex hormones, shutting down your ovaries and causing premature menopause with some or all of its symptoms: hot flushes, vaginal dryness, a loss of sexual desire and a decrease in the ability to experience orgasm. Many women are told that these responses are psychological but, as a 1992 report points out, the combination of depleted estrogen and testosterone may negatively affect all three phases of the sexual response cycle: desire, arousal, orgasm.[7] Testosterone replacement therapy is still uncharted territory in 1998, and only a few doctors are prepared to risk offering their patients small, non-virilising (non-masculinising) doses.

There is considerable controversy about hormone replacement therapy (HRT) for breast cancer patients, so doctors are also reluctant to recommend ointments containing estrogen. Ask your doctor to advise you whether or not HRT is suitable for you.

In spite of these problems, you can still share intimate moments by touching and caressing, arousing sexual desire and reaching orgasm. Breast reconstruction surgery and prosthetics can go a long way towards restoring your confidence. Much will depend on the openness with which you and your partner discuss these issues.

Men are often scared of hurting their partners. As much as they want to hug and hold them, they feel shy and awkward. The solution is simple: you must initiate the first embrace – and do so the moment you return home. It will give him confidence and reassure him that you are all right, and it will go a long way towards breaking down the barriers to maintaining the love and affection you have for each other.

PELVIC CANCERS

Ovarian, cervical, vulval, bladder and colorectal cancers involve different treatments, some producing similar responses. If the cancer has invaded surrounding tissue, surgery for cervical cancer may involve a radical hysterectomy, removing the uterus and surrounding tissues; a hysterectomy for uterine and ovarian cancer requires the removal of less tissue. If you are past your child-bearing years, surgeons will invariably remove your ovaries.

Removing your ovaries before menopause will affect hormone production, producing the same side effects – premature menopause – as chemotherapy or hormone treatment described above. In both procedures, the top of your vagina is also sealed off and does not, as some people believe, become an open tube into the pelvis.

Bladder cancer is rare in women and usually requires a radical cystectomy, the surgical removal of the bladder. Pelvic exenteration is total removal of the contents of the pelvis for large cervical cancer. Without a bladder, you will require a urinary ostomy, called a ureterostomy, an operation in which an artificial opening is made in your abdomen to allow urine to pass out into a drainable plastic bag which seals into a plastic 'face plate' attached to the skin surrounding the ostomy.

COLORECTAL CANCERS

Surgery for colorectal cancer, including cancers of the large intestine and rectum, is successful in most cases. This procedure involves removing the rectum, so your doctor will create a colostomy for you – an artificial anal opening in the colon to allow elimination of waste material from the body into a leakproof bag.

Ostomy support groups tend to be better organised than most, so find the one nearest you for more information on how to cope. If you had a healthy sex life before surgery, there is no reason for this to stop. Remember, you can continue to enjoy sex wearing an ostomy bag if you make some minor adjustments:

- Check the seal beforehand.
- Make love in the shower.
- Choose a time of day when you know your colostomy is less or not active.
- Tuck the pouch into the elastic support belt.
- Create a romantic setting: turn down the lights, open a bottle of wine – or be a devil, put a rose between your teeth.
- Wear sexy underwear, such as crotchless panties or teddies, or use a pillow or cushion to cover the pouch.

Radiation and chemotherapy for pelvic cancers can produce similar side effects to those experienced by women treated for breast cancer. Some of their side effects can affect your sex life; most are usually temporary. Here are some examples that may, or may not, apply to you:

- Radiotherapy can cause the lining of the vagina to become thin and fragile; this can be accompanied by ulcers or sore spots that take some months to heal.
- Radiation can cause scarring and so shorten or narrow the

vagina. Using a vaginal dilator or having regular intercourse can keep it stretched and open.

☞ Radiation for cervical cancer may cause your ovaries to fail and lead to a thickening of the fibres of the vagina and so make intercourse difficult. These symptoms may not occur until years after treatment.

☞ Chemotherapy, antibiotics and steroids can cause yeast infections making intercourse difficult and painful. Wearing loose cotton clothing and underwear, and using anti-thrush treatment, usually clears the problem.

Extended foreplay, the copious use of lubricants and ointments, the adopting of different positions, and a bit of imagination can help you overcome most side effects. A loving and considerate partner can make up for the problems of intimacy, even if sexual intercourse becomes difficult or impossible.

If ovarian function is affected, simple tricks like using an estrogen vaginal cream can improve lubrication and increase arousal. Half the fun is often putting in the cream!

Many cancers are hormone-sensitive, so your doctor may advise you to wait for at least two years after treatment for breast cancer before becoming pregnant. Chemotherapy and radiation to the pelvic area can often cause infertility, but no adverse effects on your sex life.

How men can overcome sexual side effects

Pelvic cancers in men include those of the colon, rectum, bladder, prostate, testes, and penis. Physical side effects are much the same as for women and include fatigue, nausea, vomiting, loss of hair. Emotional side effects include fear, depression, guilt and changes in self-image. Men often relate impotence to a loss of masculinity, producing feelings of lowered self-esteem and anxiety.

Men face many of the same issues as women following treatment for bladder and colorectal cancers, but testicular cancer, prostate cancer and Hodgkin's disease create a new set of challenges. If you plan to have a family and you are likely to experience prolonged or permanent sterility, talk to your doctor about sperm banking. It is also possible to have children through artificial insemination or IVF (*in vitro* fertilisation) after treatment if your sperm is still potent, even though you have a low sperm count.

COLORECTAL AND BLADDER CANCER

Surgery for colorectal cancer involves removing the rectum, so your doctor will create a colostomy for you – an artificial anal opening to allow elimination of waste material from the body into a leakproof bag.

Bladder cancer is more common in men than women, and also usually requires a radical cystectomy, the surgical removal of the bladder, prostate and surrounding vessels and tissue. A urinary ostomy (as described above for women) may also be necessary.

The most common side effects you are likely to experience are difficulty in achieving or maintaining an erection, or being able to ejaculate. Your doctor may suggest you use a vacuum erection device or learn to give yourself an injection – slightly painful, but very effective. Nerves often regenerate, but slowly, so your doctor may advise you to wait for up to a year before considering a penile prosthesis.

As mentioned above, there are ostomy support groups, and techniques to make a continuing sex life possible and enjoyable.

Some chemotherapy and hormone drugs lower testosterone levels, leading to reduced libido, difficulty in achieving an erection, lowered sperm count and less intense orgasms. These side effects usually wear off after treatment.

PROSTATE CANCER

Surgery for prostate cancer involves removing the prostate and surrounding vessels, often damaging the nerves in the area. A radical prostatectomy usually results in a complete inability to achieve an erection, although partial recovery is possible.

The side effects of radiation and hormone therapy depend on the extent of your disease and the intensity of the treatment. In general, they will reduce your desire for sex, and make it difficult to achieve an erection. The good news is that these symptoms usually lessen in time.

It is important to discuss these issues with your partner; better still for both of you to talk them over with your doctor and a sex therapist. There is hopefully more to your relationship than sex, and there are still many ways in which you can give each other pleasure, maintain sexual activity, and achieve orgasm. Some doctors claim they can spare nerves in surgery so their patients can still achieve erections; others believe that 'nerve sparing' surgery is risky, as it may leave some cancer cells behind. Talk it over with your specialist.

TESTICULAR CANCER
This rare but highly treatable cancer may involve surgery for the removal of one or both testicles. You may also require radiation and chemotherapy.

Unilateral orchiectomy (removal of one testicle) causes no infertility, and does not impair sexual function. A bilateral orchiectomy will cause infertility, lower desire and create difficulties in achieving erection and orgasm. Chemotherapy can cause infertility, though this is often not permanent; radiotherapy has a temporary effect on sperm production.

HODGKIN'S DISEASE
Surgery, chemotherapy and radiotherapy are usually all used to treat this extensive disease, each producing side effects to some degree or other.

Chemotherapy can often result in a shrinking of the testicles and a lowered sperm count; radiotherapy can also reduce the sperm count and, in larger doses, can cause permanent sterility. If you plan on having a family in the future, banking your sperm is a good idea. Talk to your doctor about this.

Sex is not a performance
The sexual side effects of cancer and its treatments can play havoc with your relationships if these are based on performance. Fear of rejection and disapproval can be hard to overcome, especially if you think you have to win a gold medal to prove you're back to 'normal' – and 'normal' doesn't exist any more. It is likely you will be able to continue with your sexual relationships as before, but don't despair if you can't.

As a first step, you and your partner need to accept that recovery from treatment takes time. You both need time to adjust, to talk things over and be honest with each other. You may have once considered sex the only way to express your love for your partner;

perhaps now you can discover other ways in which to relate to each other. Beyond sexual desire and excitement there lies the real possibility of discovering a love that goes beyond the physical. At the very least, your partner can offer you warmth, closeness, compassion, support, wisdom. You can still cuddle each other, engage in alternative sexual play, discover new erotic zones. Instead of making love in the old-fashioned way and regarding everything else as perverted, freeing your fantasies can help you explore the uncharted areas of your own sexuality. It takes frankness, courage and maturity, but if none of this is good enough for your partner, perhaps you need to ask what you meant to him or her in the first place.

Single people and side effects

In all situations, we cope better when we have someone to talk to, someone who will share our fears, anxieties and hopes. It can be particularly difficult to face the sexual side effects issues of cancer alone, especially if you have just started or hope to start a new relationship, and you dream of marriage, having children. But what do you say to someone who has no brothers or sisters, no meaningful relationship with their children or, as in the case of Sarah, no parents?

Sarah, an attractive young woman of 28, came to see me soon after she had completed treatment for breast cancer. Her boyfriend had deserted her when he learned of her problem; she had no idea where her parents were, had lost contact with them years ago, now did not wish to see them. We discussed various options, finally she said, 'I see a wonderful opportunity ahead of me to find out who I really am, and to define myself as an individual – not as someone else's alter ego. Some day, someone's going to have to accept me for who I really am – and the right person will!'

Talk to your doctor, ask her to refer you to a sex therapist, a psychiatrist, a counsellor. Join a support group and, when you're ready, start socialising again. Your cancer may make you feel more isolated than before, but you have to take the plunge, start life anew. At some stage, you will have to confide in a new mate, tell them the truth about what you've been through, what you can still do, what you hope to achieve, whether you can have children or not.

Life doesn't stop when you have had cancer; it goes on with a new honesty, and without any secrets.

Part Three

helping yourself,

helping others

nine

what are your rights?

'Education is what you get when you read the
fine print; experience is what you get when
you don't.'

PETE SEEGER (FOLK SINGER)

Your right to choose

Your ability to cope with your treatment, side effects and after-care depends largely on your understanding and awareness of your options – as well as those rights to which you are legally and ethically entitled.

You may believe you have no choice but to follow a course of treatment you would rather avoid, or surrender control over your life at a time when you would rather maintain your independence. But you do have choices, you do have rights, morally and legally. The doctor who suggests a course of treatment – whether it is standard or a trial – without offering you an alternative, or who fails to inform you about the possible side effects and consequences, prevents you from exercising the rights to which you are entitled.

You and your doctor need to know your rights so he can meet your needs and expectations, and you can obtain enough information to help you make an informed choice about the treatments being offered to you – whether to accept them or not, how far you wish to be treated, and how you wish to live or die.

Whose life is it – yours or your doctor's?

You are likely to feel helpless, depressed and ready to give up if you are told, or led to believe, that nothing more can be done for you. It may be true that your disease cannot be completely cured, but it is never correct to say that nothing can be done or that you have a fixed time to live. Something can always be done: you can try a new treatment, ease your suffering, improve your quality of life for however long you live. Shakespeare was right when he said that 'present fears are less than horrible imaginings':[1] the more you know, the less fearful you are likely to be.

I hope you feel encouraged rather than intimidated by this, and that the following pages help you feel more confident in the therapeutic partnership you have with your doctor. It's not just your body we're talking about, it's your life – so only you can decide what you want to do with it. I think you place an onerous burden on your doctor if you expect him to make all your decisions for you, if you say, 'Do whatever you think is right,' or ' I don't want to know. You tell me what to do.' Moreover, it has been my experience, and that of many others, that if you surrender your basic rights, you make it extremely difficult to retrieve them – or for your doctor to relinquish them – at a later stage.

Your specialist is an expert in the treatment of cancer, but it is your fears and hopes that matter, not your doctor's. It is your life that may be on the line, not his. It is important that you ask the questions I listed in the previous chapters to make sure he has presented you with the whole picture. In most countries, doctors are bound by ethical guidelines to give you information about your treatments, options, and material risks – and to answer all your questions.[2]

No doctor should ever presume that he is obliged to answer only the questions you ask. It is your doctor's responsibility to present you with *all* the facts you need in order to make an informed decision about your treatment – and give you enough time to make up your mind without forcing you into making an instant decision. Failing to meet his obligations denies you the freedom of choice that is your right – and it can cause problems, for example, with your nursing care.

Nurses are obliged to promote and safeguard the well-being of their patients, to 'act for and on behalf of patients, provide information, clarification and reassurance'.[3] They are placed in a difficult situation if, for example, after discussions with your family, your doctor has ordered that you be kept in the dark. You need the information to make choices even if this means refusing treatment, but your nurse has been ordered not to say anything. What is a nurse to do? Your nurse cannot fulfil his or her role honestly, and is likely to avoid you, if your doctor and your family believe it is in your best interests to keep you uninformed.

The best decision is the one that's best for you – not your doctor or your family. In this regard, a 1996 study reported in the *British Medical Journal* confirmed that people would prefer their doctors to respect their wishes, not those of their family, should they differ.[4]

The only way your doctor can overcome these problems, honour your rights and be at ease with his conscience, is to make all his decisions based on knowing as much as possible about you: your values, beliefs, family background, economic circumstances, moral and ethical values, your fears as well as hopes. Is it a big ask? I don't think so – not unless your doctor sees you as a brainless, organic object.

What is 'informed consent'?

Consent, by definition, means voluntary agreement with, not surrender to, the wishes of another. In a medical context, informed consent can only be given when you have been given an understanding of what will be involved in a medical or surgical procedure – and you give your permission in full awareness. Obviously, it may not be obtainable in a life-or-death emergency or where an individual is physically, mentally or legally unable to make an informed decision and requires someone else to act on his or her own behalf.

Informed consent implies no duress; you cannot be expected to be a fully co-operative patient or take an active role in your recovery if you feel you are being pressured. There are times when doctors and hospitals lose sight of this fact, and fail to appreciate that it is your consent that is important – not your signature at the foot of a form shoved in front of your nose which you are urged to sign without a proper reading. In most Western countries, including Australia, your doctor has an obligation in law to warn you of the probable known dangers and likelihood of consequences if you fail to heed his advice, but weighing up the risks is not a medical judgement – it is yours.[5]

Some doctors argue that it is not appropriate to divulge all the possible risks than can occur during or after a procedure or a trial; others contend that if all the risks *were* highlighted, no one would ever undergo surgery, take another pill, or volunteer for a clinical trial. I wonder.

A week before I took part in the trial of an experimental drug, my doctor handed me a consent form and several pages of an accompanying protocol supplied by the drug company. Each page was crammed with precise details of the treatment and all possible consequences —including death. My doctor urged me to read everything carefully before signing. By the time I signed the consent form I had read the protocol several times. I knew what I was letting myself in for, but for me the possible benefits outweighed the risks.

It isn't good enough for a doctor to furnish you only with information you have specifically requested.[6] While I was still on the drug trial program, I was asked to consider taking part in the trial of another, controversial new drug. I asked questions, and learned that it was being tested against both the drug I was currently using and a placebo. Had I agreed, there would have been only a one-in-three chance I would continue receiving the drug I was currently using, and a one-in-three chance I would receive no medication at all. I had been so gravely ill, I could see no logical reason to take part in the trial of another drug while I was already responding to the one I was on. I demurred.

Informed consent is not simply a reflection of the knowledge you have gained which has enabled you to choose the most appropriate treatment. Informed consent mirrors your awareness that being in control is preferable to feeling helpless, that exercising free choice helps you maintain your sense of freedom, autonomy and self-respect.

Your right to refuse treatment

The logical extension of your right to choose treatment is your right to refuse it, even it means your death. This is an unqualified right provided you choose to do so voluntarily, are of sound mind, and have been completely informed about your condition.[7]

Few of us want to die; we all want to live – but at what price? Some people are prepared to suffer prolonged periods of treatment no matter how harsh they are, others would prefer to allow their disease to take its natural course. Modern medical technology has created a dilemma: doctors can now keep us alive even when they know there is no cure for our condition, but the price of their actions is to deprive us of any quality of life. As Professor Lanham points out in his informative book, *Taming Death by Law*, the saving of life is an unqualified good, but 'it is for the patient to determine what condition or treatment is intolerable'. You may be in pain so unrelenting, tiredness so unrelieved, you are quietly desperate. You want the pain to stop, feel so weary you just want to let go. What do you do? What does your doctor do as he watches you suffer, but has to weigh up all the technology at his disposal against your desire to put an end to your suffering? If you are bed-ridden, in constant unrelieved pain and there is absolutely no chance of improvement, and you're just waiting to die – I believe you still have to ask yourself three questions:

1   Have I explored *every* option?
2   Has my doctor explored *every* option?
3   How realistic is my expectation that I will survive, and if it is fairly realistic, for how long might I live?

Only when you have asked yourself these questions and satisfied yourself about the answers can you really make an informed choice. If you want to refuse treatment, you need to be aware that while it may hasten your death, it will not necessarily relieve you of your suffering immediately; it may cause you even more pain and discomfort.

I believe that no one other than you should determine how much, or how little, suffering you wish to endure; no one else should be able to decide how you should live or die. You have to give your consent, either orally or in writing, to ensure that *your* wishes are met, and that your doctor is protected against prosecution if he helps you to fulfil your wishes. Your prior consent is also necessary to ensure no pressure is brought to bear on your doctor by family and friends in order to minimise *their* suffering or, even worse, to seek some personal gain.

No one can force you to act against your will as long as you are aware of what is going on. Your spouse/partner, family and friends may feel they cannot stand by while you suffer, but they have to realise that not only is it unethical to suggest that you stop treatment, it is illegal for them to assist you in any way other than to provide you with love, understanding and moral support. In no way should anyone ever you tell you, 'Do what I say!' or imply that if you don't you are 'letting down the side'. Their intentions may be good, but they will fail to achieve what they intended if they make you feel guilty and ashamed for not having the courage or willpower to live up to *their* expectations. The best they can do at this time is to open their hearts to you and let you know that whatever you choose to do is OK with them.

The healing potential of the attitude people bring into a critical situation can make all the difference between success and failure, so your family and friends need to remind themselves that *you* have to want to undergo a particular type of treatment; *you* have to feel confident it will be effective; *you* have to want it to relieve your misery; *you* have to believe that it will reverse the course of your disease. I believe they have to respect your wishes, and if they can't or won't, perhaps they have to ask themselves who is in crisis – them or you?

Research conducted in the USA in 1981 has shown that people who prematurely stop their treatment thereby reduce their chances of survival substantially – *and that most drop out because their family and friends pressured them to submit to the treatment in the first place.*[8]

Your family and friends may wish only the best for you, but it is not their willpower or discipline that will get you through this difficult time. You need to meet *your* expectations, not theirs. Making your own choices will give you the strength necessary to carry you through your struggle.

There are a number of excellent books which examine these issues in detail. I have listed them at the end of the book. I urge you to consult them. [9]

What happens when you are no longer competent?

You have a common-law right – *as long as you are competent* – to refuse treatment. This right also applies if, after you have undergone various treatments and are receiving life-sustaining treatment, you decide that 'enough is enough' and choose to be removed from a ventilator and refuse tube feedings and hydration.

It's one thing to choose to refuse treatment while you are consciously aware – it's quite another to allow yourself to be placed at the mercy of a doctor or anyone else when you are, for whatever reason, rendered *incompetent* and unable to make your wishes known. There are ways in which you can make your wishes known while you are competent, and also ensure your wishes will be respected when you are no longer competent by appointing an agent to act on your behalf. An appointed health care agent can act for you under certain circumstances, such as complete loss of ability to communicate. For example, in Australia and the USA, a competent adult, and anyone who has completed a DPAHC (Durable Power of Attorney) can stop mechanical ventilation when or if they decide they no longer wish to use it.

Laws vary from country to country, state to state, so check with your doctor or lawyer about a living will or enduring power of attorney. Most people fear *the process of dying* rather than death itself, and agonise most over the prospect of being alive and unable to communicate, or being treated as a vegetable. Taking care of this matter now will provide you with a great sense of freedom, and help you turn your attention to surviving rather than dying.

A new lease on life

You may feel uneasy or think you're tempting fate, but signing a living will or an enduring power of attorney will remove all lingering doubts about what will happen to you when you are no longer aware of what is happening around you. I don't believe anyone should actively seek to end their lives unless they are in unrelenting, unrelieved pain or discomfort, but choosing how you *don't* want to die can help you turn all your energy and attention away from death, help you focus on how you want to live.

I don't believe you can be truly life-affirming in your actions unless you recognise that no matter what steps you take to prolong your life, you will eventually die. You will never be prepared for death, no matter how many documents you sign if you believe you will live forever. Signing a living will or enduring power of attorney will not only help you come to terms with your own death while it is still a relatively distant event, it will ensure that your wishes are respected to your very last breath. The ultimate expression of freedom of choice is control over your destiny. One of the most life-sustaining actions you can take is to try to make sure your death is as close to your ideal of it as possible.

There may still be confusion about what you want, even if you have written out a living will or signed an enduring power of attorney. The more that is known about your personal set of values, the more likely your wishes are likely to be honoured when you are no longer competent, no matter where you live, whether your rights are recognised under common law or legislation or not. To make it easier for those who will have to decide what treatment to accept or refuse on your behalf, the Institute of Public Law at the University of New Mexico has devised a 'values history form'. The purpose of this values inventory is to help you review what you feel is important about your health. Questions on the form cover attitudes to life and health (e.g. what, for you, makes life worth living); personal relationships (e.g. how would you expect friends and family to support your decisions on medical treatment); attitudes to independence and self-sufficiency; living environment; religious convictions (e.g. how do your beliefs affect your feelings about illness); relationships with health professionals; general thoughts about illness, dying and death; finances; funeral plans.

Completing this form does not mean you shouldn't make a living will or appoint an agent, but it provides valuable supplementary information about your wishes and values. If you do complete it, you may wish to give copies to your doctor, your family or friends, your legal adviser.

The Resources Guide at the back of the book tells you how you can obtain a copy of this invaluable document.

A living will refers only to your extended right to refuse medical treatment; it does not apply to the discontinuation of life-supporting treatment, often referred to as *passive* euthanasia (see below). If you request someone to deliberately cause your death (*active* euthanasia), either orally or in a living will, and he or she complies, it could, theoretically, be classed as murder.

Euthanasia

Thousands of books and articles have been written on the subject of euthanasia, and it is not within the scope of this book to examine all the arguments for and against the ethics of it. However, it is an issue hard to avoid when discussing cancer. To begin with, you need to understand what certain terms mean.

Active euthanasia refers to the intentional termination of life to relieve suffering through some deliberate action.

Passive euthanasia is committed when someone omits or forgoes a life-preserving action.

Voluntary euthanasia refers to the ending of life through someone's informed request and free consent.

Non-voluntary euthanasia occurs where there is no consent and applies, for example, to the killing of an unconscious patient based on a surrogate's decision.

Euthanasia against someone's will is called *involuntary* euthanasia.

Direct euthanasia occurs when life is ended intentionally and actively as the result of a specific action.

Indirect euthanasia means allowing death to occur without a direct link between the action, intent and result. Indirect euthanasia is frequently used to describe the hastening of death by an action that is primarily intended to relieve suffering or promote some other good, but is also known to be potentially lethal – for example, the use of morphine to alleviate air hunger and distress in someone dying of respiratory failure.

You are entitled to receive, as a doctor is entitled to provide, pain-killing treatment even if this will hasten your death, but actively helping you to die is against the law and goes against guiding medical principles.[10] The Hippocratic Oath taken by doctors clearly states: 'I will follow that system of regimen which, according to my ability and judgement, I consider for the benefit of my patients, and abstain from whatever is deleterious and mischievous. I will give no deadly medicine to anyone if asked, nor suggest any such counsel.'

Everett C. Koop, one-time Surgeon General of the United States, once said that

> *There is a difference between helping a person live all the life they're*
> *entitled to and prolonging the act of dying. There is also a difference*
> *in letting nature take its course in a dying life and speeding the death*
> *of an individual by whatever means and for whatever purposes, no*
> *matter how well intended.[11]*

What do you do if you are the spouse, parent or child of someone with cancer and feel you have to do something – anything – to help the one you love because they cannot face any more pain or discomfort?

Words like 'aid-in-dying' and 'suicide' wrestle with words like 'murder' and 'self-deliverance'. The commandment, 'Thou shalt not murder' seems at odds with trying to help someone you love to die gently.

'Death with dignity' and 'the good death' mean different things to different people. Doctors think patients don't want to talk about it; patients think doctors lack the time and the training to do so. Others are cynical about the motives of their doctors. Ethicists, researchers and politicians at some emotional distance from these issues have different agendas from doctors and patients; but whose needs are crying out to be met – theirs, your family's, your doctor's, yours?

The desire to refuse treatment often leads to the ethically, and legally less clear, and highly controversial, issues of refusing life-sustaining treatment, assisted death, euthanasia (direct or indirect). These are important issues and cannot be ignored.

Is euthanasia legal?

There are many pro-euthanasia advocates who quote the legal system in Holland as the model other countries should follow but, contrary to popular belief, euthanasia is *not* legal in Holland. Through verbal agreements between the Justice Department and Royal Dutch Medical Association, most doctors will not be punished if, when asked by a dying patient to end their suffering, they meet certain criteria. The Royal Dutch Medical Association emphasises that even when they comply with these requirements it is murder, unless euthanasia is performed at the request of the patient.[12] In other countries, any type of euthanasia – pulling the plug, administering a lethal potion, and so on – is illegal.

Efforts to legalise euthanasia in the Western world have been gaining ground. Much of the motivation for it reflects a genuine desire to alleviate pain and suffering. Against this, I would argue that recent advances in more effective pain control, better management of other distressing symptoms and improved psychological and social support of the dying can alleviate suffering and reduce the perceived need to resort to active euthanasia.

There is also a growing awareness that we need to guard against the technological imperative – the pressure to use new technologies and treatments. Perhaps this implicit pressure would lessen if the emphasis on doctor education returned to the gentler and kinder, albeit time-consuming, aspects of caring for the chronically ill and the dying, listening to their fears and controlling their pain. As Dame Cicely Saunders, founder of the hospice movement in the United Kingdom, reminds us, palliative care, as defined by the WHO, is based on the understanding that a person is an indivisible entity, a physical and spiritual being. As she points out, 'The only proper response to a person is respect.'[13] In many doctor–patient relationships, indirect euthanasia – rather than yet more treatment – is the eventual outcome of love, compassion and understanding.

Euthanasia societies around the world urge their members to make sure that in each particular case no other acceptable solution to their dilemma is available. Choosing to end your life is, they argue, an irreversible decision and one that should never be taken lightly, without full and conscious deliberation, and without thinking how your actions may affect your family.

They also point out that you need to be aware how people react differently in a crisis. For example, your family may agree to follow your wishes, but when the time comes to act, they may find them hard to carry out – especially if they still hope for a miracle recovery. Your spouse/partner, family and friends need to recognise that it is not their right to make decisions about your treatment. By any definition – euthanasia, mercy killing, assisted suicide, or deliverance – pulling the plug on your life-sustaining equipment or administering a lethal potion on your behalf is *murder*.[14]

THE 'SLIPPERY-SLOPE' ARGUMENT

Much of the debate around euthanasia has centred around the 'slippery slope' argument – the view that once we accept the notion of active euthanasia (deliberately terminating someone's life) we break a general moral prohibition against killing, and there will be nothing to prevent us going further. First, there would be active euthanasia for those who request it (voluntary euthanasia), then compassionate (indirect) euthanasia for those who are unable to request it – the comatose or those in intractable pain. From there it would be only a short step to killing the mentally disabled and the mentally ill; the senile, the elderly, the mentally retarded, the chronic schizophrenics, patients with Alzheimer's disease. Furthermore, the argument goes, as the population ages and the cost of caring for the frail elderly increases, there will be a minority demand for non-voluntary euthanasia of dependent patients who lack full decision-making capacity. In such a scenario it is not hard to imagine how the non-treatment of any life-threatening condition might become routine – a not impossible prospect if cost-cutting reduces levels of care, especially for the less well-off.

Justice Rehnquist, writing for the US Supreme Court in 1997, clearly articulated the dangers that legalised assisted suicide (active, voluntary euthanasia) would pose, particularly to those who are most vulnerable: 'The risk of harm is greatest for the many individuals in our society whose autonomy and well-being are already compro-mised by poverty, lack of access to good medical care, advanced age, or membership in a stigmatised social group.'[15] Rehnquist also noted that Washington's Natural Death Act, enacted in 1979, states that the 'withholding or withdrawal of life sustaining treatment "at a patient's direction" shall not, for any purpose, constitute a suicide.'[16]

The assumption behind the slippery-slope argument is that just as you brutalise the hangman, you will do the same to your doctor. In the end, he may see the person he helps to die as just another case resolved. Experience in Holland suggests that this is a real risk. A study conducted by the Dutch government in 1990 found, that

> despite the existence of various reporting procedures, euthanasia in the Netherlands has not been limited to competent, terminally ill adults who are enduring physical suffering, and that regulation of the practice may not have prevented abuses in cases involving vulnerable persons, including severely disabled neonates and elderly persons suffering from dementia.[17]

Suicide

For some people, suicide is a way of retaining ultimate control over an intolerable situation; for others it is the only solution to chronic, unrelieved pain, untreated depression, a sense of helplessness and a feeling that they have become a burden, financial and otherwise, to their family and friends. Suicide may seem the only way out when death becomes preferable to facing life, but those who turn to suicide are usually those whose depression has not been treated, and who have not been fully informed about other options that could give them hope or alleviate their suffering.

In her book, *When is it Right to Die?*, Joni Eareckson Tada talks of the 'tempting lies the Devil whispers in our ears' in trying to persuade us life isn't worth living and death is preferable.[18] The moral legitimacy of euthanasia – and suicide for that matter – needs to be weighed up with continued existence too painful to bear on one scale, and an obligation to seek extraordinary measures to effect a cure on the other. For many people, suicide is their expression of their dilemma: they want to escape death through some miracle that will save their life, and they want to escape pain and suffering by ending their life. I believe that life demands preservation. I felt this as a moral imperative when I was desperately ill and living from one blood transfusion to the next.

In quiet moments of prayer and contemplation, I became aware that over and above my abiding optimism that a cure would be found, the decision as to whether my life was worth living or not was not mine to take. Death would have been an easy way out of my suffering, but I did not feel as if I possessed absolute title to my life or my body; I felt I had a responsibility to take care of the life that I had been privileged to receive. I finally accepted that as long as I could breathe I would do whatever I could to preserve my life. In retrospect, I felt this was the right choice, for two reasons: to pre-empt the timing of my death would have been to disturb the harmony I had struggled so long and so hard to achieve, and I wouldn't have been around to take advantage of the drug that saved my life!

As you may already have discovered, you never know how much more you can cope with until you have to. Choosing suicide as soon as you have been diagnosed with your disease or after having undergone a course of treatment may not only prevent you from testing your limits of endurance, it will guarantee you won't be around when a cure is found for your disease.

Yet I find it hard to be critical of anyone who feels that life has become intolerable, that their suffering is not an ennobling experience, and that dying by their own hand is the only way to relieve everyone around them of the burden of care. None of us has a moral right to define how anyone else should choose to die; everyone has a chosen path to follow. This applies to your family as well. You may decide that you have become a burden on your caregivers, but they may see your illness as a unique opportunity to express their love and devotion towards you: committing suicide may well rob them of a rare way in which *they* can come to terms with their own feelings towards, and their own fears about, *their* own eventual death.

You will help your loved ones start the grieving process they will eventually have to face without you if you allow them to share your hopes and your fears, and allow them the opportunity to provide you with support and comfort in your time of need. The courage of the dying is often a source of comfort and strength to the living. In my own case, my sons and my father were comforted by my will to live and my acceptance that death was not to be feared.

There is a very real danger that more and more people will choose suicide in order to overcome their fear of dying instead of coming to terms with it. In the light of this, I have come to view, with a large degree of cynicism, those who vociferously advocate euthanasia when they themselves are not facing a life-threatening disease.

It may, at first, appear to be only a semantic difference, but in law your right to refuse treatment which may save your life is not regarded in the same light as actively life-*shortening* medical treatment – whether this takes the form of assisted suicide or as a by-product of someone's efforts to relieve your pain and suffering. Refusing life-saving treatment is also not the same as attempted suicide. A person refusing the aid of artificial life-support equipment which cannot cure and causes strain and suffering is not the same as a person who wants to deliberately kill himself or herself.[19]

I believe we should not seek to hasten death – but neither should we seek to prolong it. We *do* have the right of choice. If, after serious consideration, you are convinced that suicide – assisted or otherwise – is the last, best and only solution for you, then you have to accept that the full and sole responsibility for that death is yours. Your fate is in your hands – and paradoxically, knowing you have the power to stop may give you the courage to carry on.

ten

understanding
feelings

‿

'A joy shared is doubled,
a sorrow shared is halved.'

ANON

Normal reactions

'It's malignant. There is no cure.'

I was so busy exploring treatment options in an attempt to prove my doctor's diagnosis wrong that I didn't feel the impact of his words until a week later. I was completely unprepared for what followed.

Following the shock and numbness I felt after being told my diagnosis, my sense of time became distorted. I felt as if I were floating in a fish tank looking out at the world: I could see everything but was shut off from all sounds and smells. The blue of the sky appeared lifeless, the green of the trees dull. I felt at times as if everything around me were happening in slow motion, at other times as if I were drifting without direction or purpose. Nothing seemed real. Voices came to me as from a distance. The blue of the sky seemed lifeless. People appeared to me as 'other-worldly'. One moment I was aware of them, the next it was as if they didn't exist. I felt stranded in the realisation that no one out there had any idea of what I was going through, what I was feeling or thinking. I was going to die and there was nothing anyone could do for me. I was stuck in my own head. I was on my own – disconnected, alienated, isolated, frightened.

There are many reactions that follow a cancer diagnosis: we can feel trapped, numb, guilty, confused, sad, lonely, anxious, panicky, scared. Abruptly confronted by the fear of our own death and the manner of our dying, we can be cut off from those we love and the things with which we are familiar. In a flash, our dreams and plans for the future are torn from our grasp and, like sailors in a storm, we find ourselves adrift without oars, without a compass, and unaware where the tide will take us. The despair can be unimaginable.

You can't will away your responses, and it is essential to your eventual recovery that you recognise them as normal. You also need to give expression to your moods and feelings rather than bottling them up, so they do not overwhelm you. This is important, because unexpressed emotions drain you of energy, and keep you focused on controlling them instead of directing your resources towards your recovery. You may also increase your sense of alienation and isolation if you keep your feelings locked away at a time when you need someone to be your sounding board or support. The only way through is to honour your feelings, and remind yourself that they will pass. Be gentle on yourself, even if you feel you can't keep two simple thoughts together.

Honour your feelings

You need to honour your feelings in your own way – not the way others expect you to. There will be times when you want to be alone, gather your thoughts, heed your inner voice rather than the words of others who say, for example, 'Be brave. Keep a stiff, upper lip. When the going gets tough, the tough get going. Think happy thoughts. Hang in there.' These expressions usually reflect an attempt to allay *their* anxieties, not yours, so ignore them. It can be extremely tiring to keep your responses under control as you try to follow someone else's advice to be stoical, suppress your fears and anxieties. It's normal to get upset; abnormal to suppress your feelings.

You may feel you want to protect those around you, but keeping your feelings locked in will not only increase your distress, it will add to their unease as well. If no one knows how you feel, they are likely to imagine the worst; instead of protecting them, you may have to deal with their feelings in addition to your own. You may find the process of calming others part of your duty, but you need to maintain your independence and your autonomy, so remind yourself who is the patient, who needs rest, and whose life is on the line.

This is a difficult time for everyone. Your family and friends may undergo many of the same responses as you, so they also need to honour and express their feelings, stop pretending everything is normal and trying to second-guess what others are thinking. The resulting tension can be overwhelming. You and your family will find it therapeutic to operate in a climate of honesty and openness that brings everyone together, helps everyone realise that acceptance of – not surrender to – the situation in which you now find yourself is a prerequisite to surviving it. Pretending there is no problem won't make it go away. Giving in to it will leave you no room to manoeuvre.

Modifying your reactions

Each new experience, each new response changes you. At no time is this more apparent, or necessary, than when you are faced with a life-threatening situation. The usual responses to a life-threatening disease are well documented and I will discuss them below, but this will be a new experience for you, and it will test your survival skills – particularly if you regard what has happened to you as extraordinary, and have always thought that ill health and death only affect *other* people.

To ease your way through this life-changing process, you need to change your response from 'Why me?' to 'What now? What can I do for myself?' 'Why me?' is a rhetorical question that reflects your despair, anger and frustration. 'What now? What can I do?' is an active statement that will help unfreeze you from the shock of your diagnosis, give you the voice of a survivor.

Turn each of your responses to your advantage in the same way, and you will not only reduce your anxiety but increase the likelihood of you living longer. Your disease may have been diagnosed at an advanced stage, but understanding your responses and modifying them can still give you a fighting chance. You'll find it a whole lot easier to manage the changes now taking place in your life if you try to see your problems as possibilities, your obstacles as opportunities, your stumbling blocks as stepping stones. At the very least, you will cope more easily with your fear of death and dying if you accept that death is neither a surrender nor a failure, and that if you die, you are not a victim.

Your responses to death

Underpinning all our responses are our fears and these, in turn, are based on that which threatens our survival – death. Fear of death drives us to deny it in a variety of ways to help us cope with the prospect of separation from those we love, the destruction of our ego, the dying process itself. Some people actively seek control over the manner and the timing of their death through suicide or euthanasia as a way of overcoming their panic and fear of the process of dying.

With our all-embracing belief that science can control everything, including death, we see it as an alien force we must fight at all costs instead of seeing it as a natural part of life. Doctors who view their inability to defeat death as a failure do their best to ignore it. Perhaps the clearest example of this avoidance is when those who have died in a hospital are wheeled out through a rear door, at night, so no one will see them. Some people look to cosmetic surgery in the belief that if they look young they will remain young; others turn to cryogenics to deep-freeze their bodies until a day in the future when science will, so they say, resurrect them. Everyone – including doctors – wants to forget that, on this planet anyway, the death rate is 100 per cent. It seems that only when we see that our death is no longer a distant possibility, but a closer probability, do we stop trying to avoid the issue; only then are we compelled to deal with what it is about death that we really fear.

You may have known someone who died, or even watched them die. If they were old, you may have thought, 'Well, they had a good innings.' If they died young, you may have thought, 'It's so unfair.' You may have believed that with scientific advances and improving medical care you could live a full and healthy life until you were 'good and ready', when death, hopefully, overtook you in your sleep.

From another perspective, everyone identifies with incredible rescues as if they had triumphed over death by proxy. The entire world breathed a collective sigh of relief in 1997 as round-the-world yachtsman Tony Bullimore was plucked from the icy waters of the Southern Ocean and, in the same year, when Stuart Diver was dug out, hand by hand, from the rubble of collapsed buildings at an Australian ski resort.

On average, we may see as many as a thousand deaths on our

television screens in the course of a single year. The only way we can cope is to constantly reassure ourselves, 'Oh well, it's only a movie,' or 'Thank heaven I don't live in Bosnia or some other war-torn region of the world!' Many of us distance ourselves from our fears about dying by engaging in death-defying activities: sky-diving, bungy-jumping, mountain climbing, high-speed driving and smoking.

The only two fears people are born with are a fear of falling and a fear of sudden and sharp noises. Both these fears are *life-saving*. I believe the fear of death is culturally acquired and becomes *life-denying* because of the amount of energy we use to keep it under control. Our behaviour is largely determined by our fears – from fear of failure to fear of death. A diagnosis of cancer compels us to face reality and acknowledge that it is only by coming to terms with death that we can begin to cope with life.

Do people go through stages?

Before describing the various responses people tend to experience in times of crisis, I should like to comment on the work of Dr Elisabeth Kübler-Ross, whose studies of dying patients are so well known.

In her book *On Death and Dying,* published in 1969, Dr Kübler-Ross put forward the view that dying people go through predictable stages of responses: denial, anger, bargaining, depression and acceptance.[1] Although her model has helped to identify many responses, I concur with Professor Allan Kellehear (*Dying of Cancer: The Final Year of Life*) that her theory has led many people to expect that their responses will follow a similar, predictable and linear pattern.[2] As Kellehear points out, her study was flawed: the questions were not structured, people were not asked the same questions; it was conducted on only a small group of people all of whom were in hospital, had not been informed of the seriousness of their condition, and had strained relationships with their nurses and other staff. Moreover, Dr Kübler-Ross provided only a *description* of the responses of her patients, although many people have come to regard her observations as a prescription of how they *ought* to respond. Largely overlooked by most people is Kübler-Ross's own remark that people should not generalise from her observations, her work was 'not meant to be a textbook on how to manage dying patients, nor was it intended as a complete study of the psychology of dying'.[3] The effect of this misunderstanding has been that many people – patients and their carers alike – have based their assessment of what to do next on whether patients are in a particular stage or not. This error has been compounded by the belief that unless each stage is properly experienced – and in the right order – there can be no progress to the next stage.

Going through 'stages' also implies a stop-start, on-off affair. On the contrary, our emotional responses constantly fluctuate in an unbroken and dynamic process. We tend to experience various emotions simultaneously rather than in a sequence; some may last briefly, others may last longer. You may experience a flood of responses all at once, then wonder why you do not seem to have experienced some of them. Watching your every action or statement in an attempt to determine which stage you are in can be highly stressful. Some people have greater control over their emotions than others, or believe they can control their emotions only to find they cannot. Kellehear correctly points out that if there is deemed to be only one logical and 'right' way for you to respond, and you don't follow this pattern, you run the risk of being labelled as deviant, abnormal or dysfunctional. Even worse, the implication is that there is something wrong with you. Emotions are never either black or white. Not going into denial does not necessarily imply acceptance, a state of non-happiness does not mean you're unhappy, the opposite of fear does not mean you're fearless.

Your responses are most likely to be like playing a board game: you land on a square, throw the dice, and go three squares forward. You roll the dice again and go four back. Just when you think a one will get you to your final destination, you throw a three and have to wait.

There may be similarities between your experience and those of others, but your response will be unique to you. It will be your own personal challenge. How you deal with it will determine how well you cope. Just be patient.

It's hard to accept the loss of your health or impairment of any of your physical abilities. It's even harder to acknowledge that something has been going on inside your body despite the fact that you played sport, exercised regularly and ate all the right foods. It can be equally difficult to deal with what has happened if you blame yourself for what you have done, or allowed to happen, that might have caused your illness: smoking, drinking, working with hazardous chemicals, inheriting the wrong genes. You will add to your distress if you dwell on these matters; better to direct your energy towards your recovery by acknowledging, as discussed in Chapter 5, that understanding what is happening to you is a fundamental rule for survival.

Shock

Anything unexpected can cause you to pause and look around. Shock can 'stop you dead in your tracks'. 'I almost died of shock' is a common expression. Shock is a physical reaction to the intensity of the emotion you have experienced. You may feel it as a pain in the pit of your stomach or a tightening in your chest, as if your heart has stopped.

Shock numbs your senses, shuts you down so you hear nothing, see nothing, feel nothing. You may be so overwhelmed, you cannot move and are rendered speechless. This reaction is common to everyone in a crisis, but the intensity of it and the time it takes to unfreeze will vary from person to person. When the numbness melts and you realise you have no future, your cry of grief begins. There may be a sudden rush of panic as you struggle to come to terms with an overwhelming sense of loss of life and those you love.

Fortunately, we are an extremely adaptable species, and our survival instincts so strong, that we do not remain frozen for long and are soon galvanised into action.

Disbelief

The moment shock lets go, the buzzing in your ears and the dizziness also stops, your hearing returns, your thoughts become focused. As you find your voice, you're first response is likely to be, 'I don't believe it!' Your disbelief may be just as pronounced even if you had persistent symptoms and underwent exhaustive tests before your diagnosis.

It's not unusual at a time like this to question your sanity, to say, 'I must be going out of my mind,' or 'I'm sure this is just a dream and I'll wake up shortly.'

You're not crazy. Disbelief at the loss of someone you love can last for months, but when a crisis happens to you it's unlikely to last for more than a few days. Your disbelief will evaporate, but rather than face the truth, you may use denial to create a reality to match your expectations and overcome your fears.

Denial
The most basic, primitive and natural defence against the impact of a shattering experience is to pretend that it's not happening, to repress and avoid it.

'It can't be true.'

'This can't be happening to me!'

'There must be some mistake!'

'They must have got the lab results all mixed up.'

Denial is not only a rejection of reality and a refusal to accept things, it is a means of protecting yourself against severe emotional stress by completely or partly repressing potentially painful experiences, past and present. Sociologists concur that most people confronted by a fatal illness express their denial of the situation by refusing to talk about it, being constantly cheerful or unrealistically optimistic about a possible cure.[4]

You may accept that you're ill, but not seriously ill; you may accept that you're seriously ill, but refuse to accept the diagnosis; you may accept the diagnosis, but deny that your condition is life-threatening. Even if you accept that it could be fatal, you may pretend that it doesn't bother you, and so ignore the implications and consequences.

'If it were malignant, they'd have got me into hospital sooner, so it can't be cancer.'

'If they don't give me radiotherapy, it can't be cancer.'

'They brought me into hospital to make sure it isn't serious.'

Denial would appear to be self-defeating, a most undesirable condition; but without some degree of denial we would probably be in a state of permanent paralysis. If we stopped to think about all the risks we constantly face as we drive to work, ride in a lift, or board a plane, we would never do anything or go anywhere. The citizens of Los

Angeles, for example, live in what has been called a 'delusion of invulnerability', without which the city would have been turned into a ghost town ages ago. Despite the ever-present risk of a potentially devastating earthquake, life goes on as normal.

It is unfortunate that the word 'denial' has been so abused, so dismissively used to label people as 'neurotic' and 'incapable of rational thought or behaviour'. *Temporary* denial is a normal psychological process we use to protect ourselves from our emotions, especially fear. It is an essential part of your defence mechanism, and acts as a shock-absorber, giving you time to take in the news, pull yourself together, and evaluate what you have been told.

Persistent or *continuing* denial, however, can be fatal if it means you delay in seeking medical treatment. For example, Dr Hackett of the Harvard Medical School estimates that at least 50 per cent of people who have heart attacks die before they reach hospital because they did not believe that the pain in their chest was a heart attack.[5] On the other hand, those who deny being frightened and ignore the seriousness of their condition *after* a diagnosed heart attack tend to survive coronary care more often than those who don't. This apparently contradictory state of affairs suggests that denial is most effective when it serves to engender a feeling of hope and optimism, and give you a sense of being back in control.

Controlled denial can help you channel your thoughts away from the gloomy and the frightening towards the bright and the cheerful. Watching reel after reel of comedy films may seem inappropriate at a time like this, but if it helps to cheer you up and make you feel better for a while, it can be a great boost. Controlled denial can be a lifesaver if you acknowledge your doctor's diagnosis that your condition is serious but refuse to believe the prognosis. It can also be of great help to you if you try to prove your doctor or the lab results wrong: a second or a third opinion may indeed prove that the initial diagnosis *was* wrong, or that the initial diagnosis was correct but that there is a treatment available for your condition. In the absence of any known treatment, your own creativity may help you find a solution – if not for your disease, then for yourself; but even this can't occur if you deny that you're even in denial!

Denial can be fragile, easily shattered by your anger when you see your ashen face in the mirror, find yourself receiving almost continuous blood transfusions, are offered no more treatments because there aren't any more to offer, and can no longer pretend you're not seriously ill. Some days will be harder to deal with than others, so if the best way you can face up to reality is to escape into a world of make-believe, it is your right to do so. I would suggest, however, that you employ your world of make-believe creatively rather than simply use it as a means of blocking out your fears. Use your imagination to develop your sense of optimism by constructing a new and vital framework for your life. You could, indeed, convert your existing reality into a more acceptable and potentially more life-saving one if you can see yourself as restored to health, surrounded by loving and caring people, and with a renewed purpose in life. It is up to your doctor to attend to the physical aspect of your disease, but it is up to you to attend to your spiritual and emotional well-being.

THE EFFECT OF DENIAL ON YOUR FAMILY
Denial can seriously affect the psychological well-being of your family, so it is important you are aware of the consequences of your actions – just as your family members should be aware of theirs.

Your symptoms may clearly indicate that you are seriously ill, but if you carry on as if nothing is wrong your family is going to be confused about what to do and how to support you at this critical juncture. You may believe that being positive means ignoring the reality of your condition, and that if your family members do not follow suit they are being negative, but if you expect them to join you in denial, you may find yourself isolated from the very people who care and most want to help you.

It is quite remarkable how denial can be viewed at once as both acceptable and unacceptable. It is unacceptable when our behaviour puts us at odds with a doctor or some other 'expert' who feels we are not facing up to reality or are being unco-operative; it is acceptable if, in the face of the most extreme situations, we carry on regardless and so spare everyone around us the awkwardness and embarrassment of having to talk about the issue at hand, i.e. if we allow *them* to deny the truth.

In some instances, denial by those around us may distance us so far from them that we are unable to communicate our real feelings. It is critical at this stage that you have someone to talk to, someone who will listen to you without being critical or judgmental, will hear your cries of grief, and will allow you to express them as you want.

DISPLACEMENT

Tension or stress can make us re-direct our emotions onto some other person or object. This is called *displacement*. The situation in which we find ourselves may be so difficult to bear that our best method of coping may be to try and get away from it all by doing something else, going somewhere else, focusing on some activity others may find strange under the circumstances.

Displacement can take a variety of forms: someone goes to a party the night his mother died; worried about his business, a man mows his lawn even though he had cut it two days earlier; unable to deal with a failing marriage, someone finds extra work to do at the office, or mops the kitchen floor for the umpteenth time. Some people mindlessly fritter away hours on end polishing the silver, rearranging ornaments, cleaning their spectacles; others continually dust the crockery, eat even when they're not hungry, visit the supermarket to buy one item at a time.

Keeping yourself busy and distracting yourself can give you a respite after your diagnosis, time to come to terms with it. Displacement is helpful if it reduces your stress levels, lets you channel your pent-up emotions into something of benefit to you or the community at large, for example, voluntary work in a hospital, church or other welfare organisation. Displacement is unhelpful if it persists and prevents you from dealing with your feelings, or learning to understand what is happening to you.

Anger

Anger is what you feel when you have been affronted or frustrated, prevented from doing what you want to do, when you know that your needs and wants aren't being met; when you sense that your territory – your life – is threatened, and you can no longer pretend that all is well.

You can't suppress your feelings for any length of time; when they boil over – as they inevitably will – your anger may not be directed as much at your disease as at yourself, for feeling the way you do.

Or it may be directed at others. 'Why me?' 'It's so unfair! Look at Joe. He drinks like a fish, smokes like a chimney, yet he's hale and hearty. Why me?' Anger like this reflects the resentment and bitterness you feel now you believe you've been robbed of your future. If your body has become weaker, you could feel irritable and even jealous that those around you still have their health and strength. Why has Fate singled *you* out? This feeling will be intensified if you have always considered yourself the centre around which everything else revolves.

You may feel that whereas you thought you were in control of every aspect of your life, there's now a part of you over which you have no control. There was a time, not so long ago, when you could go where you wanted, when you wanted. Now you find your freedom restricted because of physical pain, continuing treatment, a disability, or because you're just too tired.

Blame is often a key element of anger. You may find yourself directing your anger at someone or something else: God, your wife, your husband, your mother-in-law, the tobacco industry, the drug companies, food additives, pesticides. Doctors are almost always a prime target. People tend to blame their doctors if the tablets don't work, the treatment produces side effects, they fail to recover. They may even blame previous mismanagement for their current problems. As long as you believe doctors can cure every disease, you will tend to blame them rather than accept the fact that there are still some diseases for which there are no cures, some treatments that work better with some people than others.

Be patient: anger and blame, like thunder and lightning, eventually pass.

LETTING GO OF ANGER
Anger is a normal response to a changed situation over which you feel you have lost control. You can't always alter the situation in which you find yourself, but you can always change your responses. Anger is such a powerful response, it seems a pity to waste such a reservoir of power and energy.

Suppressing your anger releases stress hormones which depress your body's immune system; turning your anger on yourself is self-destructive and can put a distance between you and those caring for you; turning it against someone or something else is energy-sapping, potentially dangerous.

Channel this emotional force, and you can turn your crisis into a challenge, turn your life-threatening situation into a life-enhancing one. The most effective way of doing this is to stay focused on yourself, be aware of what you're doing at every moment. This is not being self-centred, but rather self-preserving in a time of chaos when it is essential that you try to maintain your autonomy. Instead of viewing your anger as reactive, make it active; turn the adrenaline surge it causes into an energy source to give you a powerful sense of being alive and determined to live again.

Anger and depression are two sides of the same coin, so if you fail to resolve the cause of your anger, you are bound to feel depressed. It is often pain that makes you angry, especially if you feel you can't do anything about it. Expressing your anger will make you feel better, since you will be, quite literally, releasing excess pain – physical as well as emotional. This does not mean throwing chairs or lashing out at other people – that's aggression. It's OK to yell, shout and boo at a football match; it's quite unacceptable to attack the players or the referee.

Anger, as steam trapped in a closed pot, must be released or else it will not only blow up and destroy the vessel, it may injure those close by – including you. Anger precedes grief, and as we need to grieve in order to heal, it is vital that you express your anger. As Woody Allen commented in his movie, *Manhattan*, 'I can't get angry; I just grow a tumor.'

You can, however, discharge your anger and depression in ways that won't hurt others or draw attention to you. Find an isolated place – or step into your car, close the door, roll up the windows – and scream. No one will hear you, and if they do, so what? Try beating a pillow, hitting a ball against a wall; go to the nearest driving range and belt the covering off very golf ball you can; walk until you can't take another step.

If you find that expressing your anger in these ways provides only temporary relief, you may need to examine your feelings more deeply to discern precisely what it is that is making you angry. A counsellor or psychologist can help you resolve this issue, and it is important that you do. Anger keeps you unbalanced; refusing to acknowledge it is to defer the possibility of your healing – and in order to heal you need to restore your equilibrium.

ANGER AND YOUR FAMILY

Your family can help you best by accepting that the situation in which you find yourself is very scary, and allowing you to honour your feelings. They need to be aware they may make you even angrier if they try to do too much for you. You are bound to feel as if your autonomy has been compromised if your competence is called into question, if you are told what or what not to eat, or refused medication on the grounds that you could 'become addicted'. Being patronised is hard to take at the best of times; when you're seriously ill, such behaviour is cruel and insensitive.

If you show anger, aggressive silence and sarcasm, those around you could react with hostility, but rather than show their feelings, they may avoid you. Remember, your diagnosis will have shaken them to the core, and reminded them of their own vulnerabilities. It is also not uncommon for families to feel as if they have contributed to your disease or that they could have prevented it from occurring. You can resolve the issues of anger and blame by talking about them, openly and honestly. There will be no surprises, no sudden or explosive reactions, if everyone puts their cards on the table, reveals how they feel and what they expect.

There is often a tendency among people who feel threatened to express their anger and frustration by putting a label onto the cause of their fears. You are de-personalised and much easier to handle if you are labelled 'unco-operative', 'self-centred', 'a difficult case' or 'a problem'. You and your caregivers will go a long way towards clearing the air of conflicts if you keep these basic issues in mind.

Bargaining
You may accept the reality of your diagnosis, but attempt to make a deal in order to gain more time, or to be spared the pain and other

symptoms you are suffering, by bargaining for your life with God, Fate, some force, even if you have never acknowledged its existence before. You may offer to attend church, temple or synagogue, promise to mend your ways, donate your organs, be more generous with your wealth and your affections. In many cases, people wish for an extension of time in order to attend a major event: a daughter's wedding, a grandson's confirmation, a family reunion at Christmas. There are countless stories of people who have prolonged their lives by hoping to be present at some event in the future. Medical intervention can sometimes aid the process of bargaining so more time can be gained, as in the well-known story of a woman I will call Hazel.

Hazel was in extreme pain. Apart from receiving injections every few hours, she was connected to other life-support systems. One day she told the staff that she wanted to attend her favourite son's wedding, which was due to take place the following week. She made it clear that if they helped her achieve this dream, her deepest wish would have been realised.

The doctor and nursing staff made every effort to build her up. On the appointed day, she was unplugged from her drips, helped to dress, and escorted to the car sent to fetch her. The staff waved her good-bye, most of them wondering if she would make it through the day, or return that evening. Hours later she returned, full of joy and beaming from ear to ear. Everyone was so pleased she had achieved her wish and would now die in peace. As she lay back in her bed, and as her drips were re-connected, she turned to doctor with a grin on her face, and said, 'By the way, did I tell you I have another favourite unmarried son – and that I plan to be at his wedding, too?'[6]

Some people achieve their trade-off and go on to deal after deal; they live from event to event. My late father is a case in point. Dad suffered his first heart attack at age 54 when I was sixteen. He told everyone he wanted to live long enough to see me married, something he clearly thought would happen in the distant future. Shortly after my marriage at age 25, he suffered a second serious heart attack and said that he would be thrilled to survive long enough to witness the birth of his first grandson. Dad had two further heart attacks, but bargained his way to the births of two more grandchildren and their respective high school graduations. When he died at 87, he had even attended two of his grandsons' university graduation ceremonies.

Bargaining reflects a determination to soldier on through the most difficult circumstances in order to use whatever time we have left in the most meaningful way possible. It may be true that bargaining for more time is an illusion, and that you would have lived just as long without striking any deals. It's a moot point.

Apathy

When bargaining doesn't help, you may become indifferent and adopt a 'So what!' attitude. Apathy is a state of lifelessness and lack of interest in events around you. Situations that once made you angry or happy no longer hold your interest. You may find yourself curling up to sleep, sleeping more, eating less. In psychology this situation is referred to as 'regression'. For those wishing to be of help, it can seem as if all their efforts are wasted, unappreciated.

Apathy can last for days, weeks, even months. Like a tortoise retreating into its shell to protect itself, you can find withdrawal an effective coping mechanism – it reduces the amount of input you have to deal with, and it can enable you to conserve your strength. But you need to see it as a *temporary* measure; as with anger, blame, denial, if apathy continues it can become destructive.

The best way to overcome apathy is to actively seek something that will help you unfold, turn your attention away from yourself. For example, it can be extremely helpful to become involved with your doctor in your treatment program. If you make some small effort in this direction, it won't take you long to realise that remaining in a state of apathy – far from shielding you – is actually preventing you from taking the kind of action that could positively influence the outcome of your disease.

Physical activity, such as walking or gentle gardening, will help rouse you out of your apathy and soothe you if you're also feeling irritable. If you are physically unable to do anything, ask someone to take you for a drive, switch on music for you, play re-runs of your favourite movies, preferably the humorous ones. The best therapy of all for apathy is talking – especially to someone who is prepared to listen, someone who knows what it's like to feel the way you do. Your best source of finding someone like that is to attend a support group, so check the Resource Guide at the back of this book.

Guilt

A sense of guilt usually strikes us when something goes wrong and we feel we could have done something more to prevent it from occurring, but failed to act. It would be unusual if you did not feel guilty and blame yourself for refusing to attend to the lump in your breast, the pains in your chest, the cough that would not go away. Feeling guilty is an unhelpful response if, instead of trying to regain control of your life, you put it in further danger. A man I once counselled almost lost his life because of this.

Brendan was diagnosed with leukemia but told his doctor and me that he was going to cure himself with alternative, non-medical therapies. For months I listened with a sense of *déjà vu*, recalling my own history, as he related all the various regimens and diets he was following. His condition worsened, and when I suggested he return to his specialist, he admitted that he felt ashamed to tell his doctor that he should have listened to him, and now felt he couldn't face him. I urged him to get medical help, but his sense of guilt still held him back until a week later a severe infection with high fever forced him to call his doctor. Brendan subsequently underwent intense chemotherapy and recovered, but as he later said to me, 'I was such a fool, I nearly died.'

Guilt can also have ill effects if it makes you feel inferior so you withdraw; you could prevent yourself from receiving attention when you most need it if you feel so unworthy of help. Those caring for you need to be sensitive to these issues, and try to make sure you are not left on your own too much, while acknowledging that at times you may want time out in order to sort out your thoughts, reflect in solitude, be at one with yourself.

You may feel guilty because you didn't fulfil your potential. You may feel that your disease is a punishment for past sins, real or imagined. You may take the blame in order to rationalise the dilemma in which you find yourself. In the absence of finding an obvious external cause, you may decide you deserve the blame for your condition. As Dr Ernest Becker points out in his Pulitzer Prize-winning book, *The Denial of Death*, as illogical as it may seem, in this state of mind it's easier to cope with your fear of death if dying is the only way you can expiate your guilt.[7]

Blame and guilt can be imposed on you by others. You may be told that if you wish to recover you must reduce your stress levels, think positively, or pray to God for forgiveness. Of course, if your condition deteriorates, even temporarily, you are likely to feel even more distressed, even more guilty and, as in Mary's case, lose your will to live.

Mary, a woman of 28, was diagnosed with breast cancer. Her cancer was not hormone-sensitive, so she could not be treated with hormone therapy; she had a mastectomy. She appeared to be doing well, but a scan some months later revealed that her cancer had recurred. Her specialist put her on the trial drug, Taxol; further scans suggested it had made her disease regress, until an event took place which set her back on her heels.

Mary's parents, devout Greek Orthodox, were distressed that their only daughter had 'lost religion'. They badgered her to attend church, told her repeatedly that her disease was punishment for not living at home 'as a good daughter should'. She refused to take their medicine, took Taxol instead and was improving until, at the behest of her parents, a priest visited her and told her, 'Unless you pray for forgiveness, the Devil – the cancer – will take you.' Mary searched her heart, but found nothing she had done was so bad she had to repent, yet the priest's words haunted her. The situation worsened as her parents' admonitions continued.

Mary died a few months later, broken-hearted, her relationship with her parents unresolved.

The only way out of your dilemma is to stop dwelling on the past and to give your life the value and respect it deserves. You can do this by assuming responsibility for all your future actions, and by starting to believe in yourself. If you believe you are worth saving, so will everyone else; if you make the effort, so will they. With your life on the line, you have everything to gain and nothing to lose.

Depression

Depression is loosely used to describe a whole range of emotions that reflect both how you feel and how others believe you are feeling: discouragement, inability to sleep or communicate, loss of energy, poor appetite, apathy, having the 'blues', brooding, grief.

We are moved to tears and feelings of sadness by many events in our lives, become depressed when this mood persists. Our words reflect our physical response to depression and despair when we say we feel choked and unable to catch our breath, have a weight or band around our chest, feel down in the mouth, are down in the dumps or in the depths of despair.

Life is essentially about relationships, so when we realise we can no longer make a difference to our relationships or find decision-making and self-control taken away from us, we feel discouraged and hopeless. The resulting devastating sense of separation and isolation can actually hasten our death.

The inability to resolve this condition has, appropriately, been referred to as the 'giving up – given up' complex. When people say, 'I wish I were dead' or 'I've had enough', their remarks often become self-fulfilling prophecies.

Depression, loss and grief

Depression may overtake you when you realise that all your prospects and expectations, the legacies and memories you thought you would leave behind, may also be lost. You may fear that the knowledge and the values that gave your life meaning will be lost or forgotten by those you leave behind, and that you yourself will, in time, also be forgotten. Some of the most profound fears you are likely to encounter will be the fear of loss of control, loss of identity, and loss of the things you have striven for in your life.

It's also normal to feel depressed as a consequence of your grief over the loss of your health and strength, your role as breadwinner, homemaker, teacher or parent, your freedom of movement, your job and the companionship of workmates, financial security. Perhaps you had made preparations for your family's future care and believed that they would be secure, but now you are forced to sell some of your possessions, even your home, because of medical and hospital expenses. You may have defined yourself in terms of your usefulness to others or enjoyed a position of authority or some standing in the community, but now feel devalued because you are dependent on others, have become a financial burden, and no longer have a vital role to play.

We express our sadness through grief, when we lose someone or something we love. Grief is a universal and basic response to loss. It is normal and natural. Over and above the racking despair we feel within, the most common outward signs of our grief are crying, difficulty in breathing, apathy, tiredness, loss of appetite, insomnia, loss of sex drive and disorientation. Mourning is the acceptable public face of grief, yet we are often prevented from expressing grief at our own expected loss of life. The situation is caused, and made worse, by people's tendency to avoid or withdraw emotionally from those whom they believe to be dying. In our desperate attempts to avoid such rejection, we repress the very emotions we need to express. We find ourselves compelled to put on a brave and cheery face, pretend that all is well. The result is yet another retreat into denial, another lost opportunity to maintain an honest relationship with those around us.

Cancer, like other life-threatening situations, brings deep-buried, long-unresolved issues to the surface and makes them more apparent. For some people, the realisation that time is short can overwhelm them with depression and grief; others feel despair when they realise that their bodies will never be the same again. It would be unusual if you did not experience grief at your loss of identity and self-image if your body has been disfigured as a result of surgery for facial, breast, testicular, prostate or bone cancer.

DEPRESSION AND PAIN

Pain and the side effects of treatments can also make you feel extremely depressed and lower your morale to the point where you're not sure whether it's worth putting up with all that discomfort. Losing weight rapidly, shedding hair, finding nothing appetising enough to eat, realising you have little or no control over your body functions, make you feel you've lost wholeness and control of what is happening to you. Depression can be exacerbated if treatment occurs over an extended period and is accompanied by ongoing discomfort and invasive procedures.

It's a vicious cycle, as depression itself produces very real physical symptoms. Apart from those I mentioned earlier, you may feel so tired you collapse into bed but then can't sleep; or, you may sleep longer, but still wake up tired; you may feel as if you can't look at food or can't stop eating. You may find you have no energy. You may feel worthless, find it difficult to think and concentrate. Trivial things you once ignored now irritate you. In situations such as this, some people even contemplate suicide.[8]

Some aspects of depression *can* be alleviated at a practical level. Your doctor may prescribe a short-term anti-depressant or a sedative to help you sleep. Pain prevention instead of pain control can greatly improve your quality of life. Hair loss due to chemotherapy is not permanent, so wearing a wig can do much to restore your confidence. Breast and limb prostheses, cosmetic surgery and make-up can work wonders for your self-image. You are much less likely to feel depressed or unhappy if you are free of discomfort and provided with relief for your pain.

Your concerns about the welfare of your parents, your children or your spouse can usually be remedied. There are welfare and aid organisations who can help (see the Resource Guide at the end of this book), and you'd be surprised at how many friends – even sometime-friends – will rally to your help. They may not appear forthcoming for fear of intruding into your space, or because they feel your immediate family members are managing well enough. Of course, if you or your family never ask, your friends will never know. They may, in fact, be waiting for a cue from you. Your failure to ask because you're unaccustomed to asking for help, or feel that this will place a burden on them, may well deny them the opportunity to be of assistance at a time when they genuinely want to help.

Letting go of depression

Depression and anger are often linked. Some people respond by being angry, and if this response fails to solve the problem, such as pain, they become depressed. Others seem to bypass anger and go straight to depression. Unresolved depression usually manifests itself as a sense of resignation, when you finally feel you no longer have control over anything and adopt a passive stance, wait for things to happen, have lowered self-esteem and let other people make your decisions for you.

I cannot emphasise strongly enough that this is not the time to hide your feelings, to suppress your tears or keep a 'stiff upper lip'. You may believe that people will consider you weak or cowardly if you don't appear brave and calm, but all you will succeed in doing is to make yourself more uptight and keeping others more at a distance.

Men were – and still are – taught from an early age that 'Boys don't cry' in the long-held belief that by repressing their feelings they will become emotionally tougher and more resilient – hence 'macho'. It has been my experience that in the face of a life-threatening disease, most men continue to act tough but deep inside experience even deeper emotions and fears than women. When you cannot reveal your feelings, your anguish is magnified.

The most effective way of lifting your depression is not to wait for things to happen, but to speak your mind, say out loud whatever feelings you are experiencing. Expression cancels out depression, tears wash away pain and anger. As psychologist Arthur Janov reminds us, if every cancer cell reflects an unshed tear, then the shedding of tears can be the start of the healing process.

Regaining control of your life at this time is essential if you want to break the gridlock in which you find yourself. You may feel there is no one close to you to whom you can speak and trust with your feelings, so seek the help of a professional therapist, counsellor, psychologist or psychiatrist. You don't need the company of doomsayers, but you do need someone who will give you moral support without judgement.

Fear

There is an old saying, 'Worry is like a rocking chair; it keeps you busy, but it gets you nowhere.' Instead of focusing on your anxieties and your fears, you need to make a plan, set a goal and, as in any process, realise you have to take the first step. Regaining your composure and starting the healing process begins the moment you start making decisions for yourself – and acting upon them. Your fears may hold you back, so it is worth looking at some of them. By recognising them, you will improve your chances of dealing with them.

Remember that our fears, like our responses, may overlap, tumble into each other, so we experience a kaleidoscope of ever-changing emotions. We rarely, if ever, go through stages of responses emotion by emotion, fear by fear.

FEAR OF CHANGE

Change is both challenging and daunting, full of promise, replete with fear. Change can keep us chained or set us free. Change can be daunting and overwhelming when it is unexpected, caused by events beyond our control. Such change brings with it fear of loss – loss of a once-certain future, of financial security, of our perception of ourselves as a healthy person, loss of mobility and independence. The ultimate fear of change is that of separation – from relationships, from those we love, from life.

FEAR OF TREATMENT

We all would have less difficulty facing our disease if we did not fear its consequences in terms of side effects, pain and, finally, death itself.

You may know someone who had a serious disease, and accompanied them while they underwent treatment. You may recall their responses, now fear you will suffer as they did.

Your fears may, or may not, be unfounded. The side effects of treatment can cause extreme distress when they produce symptoms such as nausea and vomiting, mouth ulcers, baldness and rashes. The after-effects of surgery can result in the loss of a limb, a breast or some other organ; or in the wearing of a prosthesis or colostomy bag, or being confined to a wheelchair. One of the most profound fears relating to treatment is that on one hand treatment will result in pain, and that on the other hand no treatment will result in pain. All these fears can be rationalised if you believe the treatment will be successful, that you'll one day say, 'Well, it was hard, but it was worth it.'

As I discussed in Chapter 8, there are now drugs that will control most side effects, new ways in which you can retain your physical self-image through advanced technology in prostheses and cosmetic surgery. Old attitudes towards the control of pain are changing and there are few instances when your comfort is relegated to second place. There may be occasions when treatment will not be life-saving but will be life-preserving. There may be times when treatment will make no difference to the outcome, but will alleviate pain. I believe the only way to overcome your fears is to discuss them with your specialist. It is only when you know what to expect that you can deal with them. The importance of your doctor telling you the truth about your condition was never greater than at this time.

Your fear of treatment may be based on what you have heard about chemotherapy and radiotherapy, so I urge you to read about them in Chapter 7. It is unfortunate that many people who could be effectively treated with these methods turn away from them simply because they do not understand them.

FEAR OF RECURRENCE

The treatment has stopped. Suddenly you're in limbo. Questions race through your brain.

'Did the treatment work?'

'How long have I got to live?'

'What happens next. Will my cancer come back?'

You would be most unusual if you were not afraid that your disease will recur or that it will progress – all the more so if you receive ongoing treatment or undergo repeated examinations.

Your anxiety may be fuelled by your desire to make the most of life while your family urges you to take it easy, or because you want to take it easy and your family urges you to get back to normal. You may have spent some time coming to terms with dying only to find you now have a new lease on life, as I did. You may be a little nervous about returning to work or taking up a new challenge while the fear of a recurrence still lurks at the back of your mind.

You stand a better chance of conserving your energy and improving your quality of life if you keep reminding yourself that your disease may *not* recur, that it may *not* progress. This doesn't mean you won't have moments of uncertainty, or that you won't experience some of your previous responses. It is important you remind yourself how things were before your diagnosis, how you felt good on some days but down in the dumps on others, how you coped better on some days than on others.

Remember, your reactions are normal, that feelings come and go. All you need to do to retain your sense of balance is to do what I call *life-surfing* – riding the highs and the lows of your emotions, knowing that neither one is permanent. You stand a better chance of survival if you take over the events in your life instead of waiting for them to overtake you.

What happens if your cancer does return, or if you get another, different cancer, as I did? For those who have carried on as if

nothing had happened, a recurrence usually comes as a shock, followed by even more intense reactions, an even deeper sense of
depression often leading to resignation with statements like, 'If only
I had done this or that.'

This did not happen to me. As many others before me had done, I
saw my initial disease as an opportunity to extract meaning from life,
rearrange my priorities, and follow my dream. My second diagnosis
came as a surprise rather than a shock; I was disappointed rather than
angry. As for bargaining and denial, I had long realised that they
were not my ways of coping. I found myself accepting the situation
sooner – and with it found a deeper sense of the sacred, a pervading
sense of humbleness, a renewed sense of calmness, the realisation that
no matter how confident or self-assured I might have felt as a result
of winning the first round, the ultimate choice of life and death was
not mine, that what really matters is what we choose to do between
our birth and our death, that life is a fragile, beautiful gift.

Instead of flailing around as I did the first time, I viewed my situation like a game of tennis, realised that even though I could, and
would, win several games, I could never hope to win the match. I
realised that as long as you believe you can win one more game, you
will find the strength to keep going; as long as you believe that you
defeat death when you defeat a disease, you stand condemned and
bewildered before a mightier opponent.

FEAR OF ABANDONMENT

You may fear that because you are seriously ill, your caretakers –
your family, doctors and medical staff – will abandon you.

The roots of this fear lie in early childhood. As long as we were
loved and our needs were met, we felt safe from harm, but when our
cries went unanswered, we were gripped with fear – the same fear
we carry through life that no one will hear us. We all have needs, the
strongest of which is to be loved. If this need is not met, we feel abandoned and insecure, spiritually or physically.

Emotional abandonment occurs when your doctor, with or without
the connivance of your family, stops regarding you as a competent
person and withholds the truth of your disease from you. This decep-
tion is compounded when, out of your fear of losing the support of

your caretakers, you learn the truth and then become a co-conspirator in pretending you don't know the truth. Emotional abandonment also occurs when your caretakers feel there is no point in sharing anything with you because your prospects of survival are poor, or because they feel guilty or embarrassed that they have been spared. Illogical as it may seem, they may even feel angry that in your dying you will be deserting them and so, to protect themselves, they desert you first.

Physical abandonment is more obvious. Some people may stay away because your appearance may have changed, others because visits to hospitals bring back memories of their own past experiences. Many people keep away because they simply don't know what to say. You may already have noticed how awkward and uncomfortable some people are when they visit you. Your sense of alienation is bound to increase when people visiting you start doing any of the following:

- ☞ avoid using the word 'cancer';
- ☞ spend more time talking to the person in the next bed, watching the television screen, eyeing the nurses;
- ☞ tell you about *their* illnesses, show you *their* scars, top your complaints with theirs;
- ☞ give you their unsolicited opinion of your doctor, or tell you they know a doctor who's smarter than yours;
- ☞ spend their time in another room or in the corridor talking to someone else – when you thought they were visiting you;
- ☞ sit in silence. This can be particularly distressing, as you may wonder, 'What do they know that I don't know?'

Abandonment by default takes place when you are passed from one doctor to another for different treatments. This can be particularly stressful when you become unsure whether your GP, surgeon, haematologist and oncologist are acting in concert – say when one of them orders one medication or treatment and someone else orders another, or when each of them gives you a different answer to the same question.

The most chilling aspect of abandonment can occur if your condition does not respond to treatment and your doctor regards this as his or her personal failure. Afraid to confront his own fear of failure as well as your possible disapproval, he may make his visits shorter and even stop coming, not answer your telephone calls and, when he does visit, keep at a distance.

Hospital staff abandon you when your bed is placed furthest away from the nursing control room, your call for help is the last one answered, and you aren't taken seriously when you complain of pain. There is no excuse for such abandonment but, sadly, there is little you can do about it. Fortunately, the attention provided by nurses is often selfless, caring and attentive. Some hospitals also offer pastoral care services and, together with other welfare organisations, regularly call on a dedicated group of volunteers who will visit and sit with you. Most volunteers once faced a life-threatening disease themselves, so they can appreciate what you are going through. It is not uncommon for volunteers to develop firm and enduring friendships with the people they visit.

FEAR OF BEING ALONE

The fear of abandonment reaches a climax when you are surrounded by loving, caring people, yet feel lonely, or when you find yourself in hospital, away from your familiar surroundings, and fearful that you will die alone.

People may tell you that they understand and sympathise with the way you feel, but when you are in pain or depressed, the feelings you have are yours, and yours alone. You may find it helpful in coming to terms with this response if you realise there is a difference between loneliness and being on your own.

There are many times in our lives when we feel the need to be on our own, when we want 'time out' to sort out our thoughts. To be on your own is unlikely to cause you fear if you have a comfortable sense of 'self', a sense of purpose. But you may feel very lonely if you have relied on other people to give meaning to your life, or have depended on the company of others to fill your time and are now afraid you will no longer see them. Loneliness overtakes you when you feel you are the victim of events around you or out of touch.

You can open the door to new possibilities, and raise your potential to become a survivor if you view yourself as worthy, and accept that loneliness can usually be offset by the support of caring and loving people. You may feel that asking for help or company is a sign of weakness, but it can be a lifeline, so ask for it – especially if your treatment is going to last for some time. Your family, friends and doctors are not mind-readers, and are unlikely to appreciate your fears and desires unless you tell them. If you need their help, ask.

Sadness brought on by loneliness and isolation can be overcome through companionship, through someone holding you or talking to you. You can also combat your loneliness by accepting you are who you are, and that you occupy a unique place in this universe.

Acceptance and resignation

Do you accept your doctor's diagnosis and prognosis, or do you acknowledge the diagnosis and refuse to accept the prognosis? Are you resigned to your fate, or do you accept it? There is a difference.

Resignation comes when you say, 'What's the use?' or 'I'm tired of fighting,' when you see your disease as a multi-limbed monster that will destroy you no matter what you or your doctors do. Resignation comes when you find the thought of a struggle so daunting and energy-sapping that you give up before you even start. You're one step away from waving the white flag of total surrender when you say to yourself, 'I'm going to die anyway, so what's the use of putting up with all that treatment and all that pain?'

Acceptance, on the other hand, is when you turn 'Why me?' into 'Why not me?' and realise that instead of wasting your energy in a power struggle over your disease, you can use your inner resources to focus on those things that give meaning to your life.

Acceptance entails making the best of a situation over which you have no control; resignation is to capitulate to it by adopting a wait-and-see attitude. Many survivors have discovered that the miracle of healing begins when you stop trying so hard to do something about your disease, and start working towards doing something about yourself and for yourself. You can do this if you accept the spirit of the saying, 'God, grant me the serenity to accept the things I cannot change, the courage to change the things I can, and the wisdom to know the difference.'

It takes great courage to move into this state of mind at a time when those around you are expecting you to 'show fight'. You will experience a feeling of calmness and renewed strength the moment you decide to make your own choices, deal with all the unresolved issues in your life, complete all the unfinished business you kept putting off until now, acknowledge that suffering and death are part of life, accept that you have to die at some time – but not necessarily when your doctor says you will.

In some cases, acceptance only occurs when you realise that your disease has not responded to treatment, or that your previous coping strategies have not worked. This may lead to such a desperate sense of urgency that you become irrational, race hither and thither to find a cure. I urge you to resist this, rather take note of the saying above. You may find it easier to regain control of your life if you let go of all your anger and despair, accept that it is inevitable and OK that you will die, but in the meantime make the most of your life. This was certainly true for me. My fear of death vanished as instantly as if I had poked my finger into a soap bubble the very moment I accepted that life is forever, death the key to immortality. Freed of my awesome and gut-clenching fear of death, I gained a new lease of life. Many others have achieved this. I believe you can do the same.

Success lies in meeting the challenge. Death can never be overcome, but if, between now and then, you give it your best shot, you'll be the hero or heroine of your own play. Moreover, you'll leave a legacy that's priceless: by overcoming your fear of death you will give others permission to enjoy and live their lives without fear.

Responses you can expect from family and friends

Many of the responses you experience following your diagnosis will apply, in varying degrees, to your family and friends, but there are others you can expect.

The responses of your family are potentially the most difficult to face. This is particularly true if you believe it is futile to pursue a particular treatment and want to be left alone, but they, fearful and anxious about money matters, the children and their own security, attempt to coerce you into it. Equally, you may be determined to try anything that could give you a chance of recovery, but they take what your doctor has said at face value, are completely pessimistic about the outcome, and attempt to discourage you. It is important to realise that they may not respond in the way you expect, and this can be shattering if it means that you suddenly find yourself left to your own devices and robbed of moral support.

It would be unusual if some of your family and friends didn't question the accuracy of the diagnosis, your choice of doctor, the appropriateness of the treatment, and raise the issue of alternative treatments. They may be religious and convinced that you need to renew your faith, or look for some deep psychological reasons for the cause of your illness. They may refuse to face the facts and seek out the opinion of doctor after doctor in order to find someone who will deny the diagnosis and the prognosis. They may pester your doctor to lie to you, tell you it is less serious, and question his ability. In the face of the cold truth, they may retreat into denial, even deep depression, at least for a while.

They may try to carry on as if nothing has happened, or they may imagine your condition is worse than it is and start mourning in anticipation of what they believe is your inevitable, and perhaps imminent, demise. This can be particularly distressing if they are overwhelmed by separation anxiety and push you away in order to protect themselves. This is what happened to Jack, a friend of mine, a teacher, who was diagnosed with leukemia.

A few months after his diagnosis, Jack's symptoms became worse and he was admitted to hospital for his first round of chemotherapy. He later returned to work, but when he found that he tired easily, had persistent headaches and could no longer work a full day, he resigned. Fortunately he had taken out insurance many years earlier, so he and his family were assured of a steady, albeit lower, income for the foreseeable future. Within a few weeks, his wife found herself a job, saying they needed the money and that she wanted to take care of her future. Jack was distressed at her attitude, but said and did nothing. A few months later, as he began to respond to treatment, she spurned him, saying, 'I can't sleep with a dying man.' Jack was crushed; he felt he was being treated as if he were already dead, part of a closed past. A few days later, he found an apartment to rent, and ended his marriage. Jack survived his cancer, built a new life for himself, found a new partner.

Many people will rush to your aid with offers of help of one sort or another. You could have problems if they see you as a victim or someone who is no longer competent, and decide they know what's best for you. You may need to remind them that your survival depends on understanding, theirs as well as yours, and that their taking care rather than taking *over* is what you prefer. The way to overcome present or potential difficulties is to explain to everyone how you feel and tell them about (or get them to read) the responses discussed earlier in this chapter. Also tell them that if either of you shows anger towards one another, it is not personal, rather it is an expression of your or their fears or depression. Communication is the key, as it always is.

Your family and friends may be surprised at how long it takes them to recover from the news, for their reactions to settle down, their equilibrium to return. Their recovery may take even longer if other well-meaning family members or friends push them to get over it, and urge them to get back to normal as quickly as possible. Grief counselling, open family discussions, and acceptance that everyone is affected in an individual way, will go a long way towards normalising the situation. It is essential you recognise this. You may feel angry or upset if one of your friends does not visit you as often as you would like, your once-buoyant partner weeps a lot, and the aunt you once regarded as 'the practical one' has taken to visiting clairvoyants. People who are nervous become silent or garrulous, depressed or agitated. Many resort to jokes, particularly black jokes which are an almost universal antidote (laughing in the face of death) to the fear of dying. You cannot predict how anyone will respond.

General responses you can expect from your children

The way in which your children cope will depend on their temperament and ages as much as on your behaviour. Be on the lookout for continuing and uncontrolled misbehaviour, or a complete absence of any show of feeling, chewed fingernails, crankiness, changed sleeping and eating patterns. You may need to seek professional help, particularly if your younger children's behaviour regresses so they forget their toilet training, have nightmares, and start wetting their beds.

They will find it easier to accept that their behaviour is OK if you tell them there is no such thing as a right or a wrong response – for example, they may laugh at your bald head. Also, in this time of great uncertainty, don't try to stop them from talking, even when they are sobbing; hug and hold them whenever you can.

Teenagers are just as vulnerable as younger children as they strive to maintain their balance between the world of a child and that of an adult, struggle with hormonal changes and their fear of losing you. Some may rebel and regress, others may take on more responsibility and grow up too quickly, still others will continue as if little has happened. Some children cope better when left alone, so let them, but make sure they don't withdraw completely from their normal home and school routine. Distractions may help for a while – and can be helpful to both of you – but they tend to be short-lived. Provided they are old enough, asking children to help in a particular task can empower them and give them a sense of being able to do something rather than helplessly sitting around. And, no matter what their age, take your children shopping for their favourite foods; they'll find it emotionally and physically satisfying.

Signs you are less likely to pick up include crying into their pillows at night, taking long walks, getting into fights with kids at school. They may resent seeing their friends going on outings, or watching people living apparently normal lives on some of their favourite television programs. More obvious signs that your teenagers are not coping include lethargy, anorexia, hallucinations, insomnia or extended absences from home. Most of these problems can be dealt with if you accept that they are probably linked to your condition indirectly. You will make it easier for them to stop pretending they are coping or are unaffected if, in spite of your condition, you reveal you are alert, and sensitive to their feelings. There is no magic formula to help them overcome their anxieties except for them to acknowledge their feelings openly and honestly, realise that in time they will pass, and remember the words of Rabbi Earl Grollman, who says in his sensitive book, *Straight Talk About Death For Teenagers*, 'You can't heal what you don't feel.' [9]

Over and above those described earlier, the responses of your children could include some or all of the following. Bear in mind that there is no predictable sequence in which they will occur, they may be brief or last some time, and they can occur all at once or far apart.

Shock

Shock can result in a withdrawal into silence or screaming outbursts, but it is more likely they will feel neither pain nor anger. They will almost certainly feel as though they're moving in a dream, just as you did when your doctor told you of your diagnosis. When 'words are weak/the fitting truth to speak' is a warm embrace or a hug, and allowing them to do the talking can be extremely helpful and comforting – no matter how old they are.

Disbelief and denial

Just as you found it hard to believe what was happening to you, so will your children. Depending on their age – and therefore their level of imagination and their ability to picture their own death – they will probably pretend everything is all right, even talk or carry on as if they had not heard what you said. They may wake up in the morning and forget for a while what you told them – then feel guilty because they forgot.

In an attempt to deny what you told them, they may refuse, for example, to attend school or perform a chore they previously did without complaint, and act as if they don't care a hoot. This is not the time to pretend that everything is OK. It isn't. Your understanding, gentleness and love is what they need. Now, more than at any other time, but within tolerance levels, let them set the agenda. In a day or so, they will realise you are still very much with them, will want to carry on as before, and accept normal discipline.

Guilt

Young children believe they have magical powers and that what they wish will come true. It is not surprising, therefore, that if you fall ill soon after they have had bad thoughts about you, they're going to believe that they caused your disease.

Conversely, if you ever said something like, 'Your behaviour will be the death of me' and then you became ill, they may feel an overwhelming sense of blame, terrified that you will die. You may think this is uncommon and does not apply to your children, but to ensure they do not suffer depression or carry a sense of guilt with them through life, it is vital you assure them that your disease is not their fault.

Guilt does not only apply to younger children. Older children may feel they should have done more for you in the past, and now don't know what to do. They may also feel guilty when, without realising it, they find themselves laughing out loud during a television program, then remember that you are seriously ill. You need to tell them it's OK.

ANGER

Frustrated in their desire to return things to the way they were, children may re-direct their anger in many ways. They may refuse to comply with the simplest request, shout, break their favourite toys, slam doors. They may hit their brothers and sisters for no apparent reason, make insolent remarks to their teachers, and even resort to stealing. Arrogant and hostile behaviour is often a sign of repressed anger.

Your children may be so angered at the way in which their lives have been changed while everything else around them seems so unaffected that they may refuse to take in the beauty of nature, listen to their favourite music or play sport. In moments such as this, your child's cry of grief may come out as, 'I hate you! I hate you!', directed at everyone in general and no one in particular.

At this most difficult stage, you need to show your love and understanding, rather than your criticism. You may also find it helpful to re-direct their anger by providing them with something to strike, such as a punch-bag or old pillow, or suggesting other useful or playful activities that don't hurt anyone. Provide your younger children with blocks, crayons and colouring books, cardboard boxes to build or smash. Get your older children to clean cars, assist you in planting bushes or pruning fruit trees. Do things together, watch TV, play a board game, go to a movie, tell them to invite their friends over.

DEPRESSION

Children may express depression by wanting to stay in bed, refusing to attend school, and crying. At school, they may sit and stare into space during lessons, fail to do or hand in homework, or sit on their own in the playground during breaks. Insensitivity by their teachers to these responses will only make matters worse.

Watch out for grief that is delayed, prolonged or even absent, and take note of signs of anorexia. As with the other responses, your love and attention will help you both through this difficult time. Your attitude towards your disease, particularly your honest expression of your feelings, can lift their mood, but if despite your best efforts their moods continue, get professional help as soon as possible.

GRIEF

For many children, the news of your disease will be the same as if you had already died, and their grief no less intense than that of an adult. Children often appear to get over things more quickly, but depending on their ages and levels of understanding, their grief may lie buried for a considerable amount of time, then surface as some new experience arouses it.

At a birthday party, for example, your children may ache and feel envious of other children when they notice that they are accompanied by their parents, and you are absent being in hospital or recovering from treatment. They may feel alienated when their teacher asks the class to talk about their recent vacation, and they spent it visiting you in hospital. Finding it hard to verbalise or express their feelings, younger children can act out of character for a while, so be patient – and remind them how much you love them.

Remember, expect the unexpected from family and friends no less than from your children. Your responses will affect them, and vice versa. This is a time for everyone to honour each other's feelings, heed the words of the poet and thinker, Goethe:

> *If we take people as they are, we make them worse.*
> *If we treat them as if they were what they ought to be,*
> *We help them to become what they are capable of becoming.*

eleven

caring and support

*'The only thing we have in front
of death is friends.'*

C REE I NDIAN SAYING

Expect the unexpected

Home looks different when you've been diagnosed with cancer.
Before it looked familiar, made you feel comfortable, and was the
place where you were surrounded by your family and friends as they
focused their love and care on you. Now it looks like someone else's
house, makes you feel uncomfortable because you are in a different
and possibly dependent role, and is the place where you feel like a
stranger trying to fend off the hospitality being bestowed upon you as
people start arriving at your door, calling you on the phone and sending you baskets of fruit, bouquets of flowers and racks of get-well
cards.

Friendships can be transformed too. In my own case, people I had
thought I could count on stopped calling; whereas strangers provided
unexpected help, and casual acquaintances became good friends. You
may be angry or disappointed at the response of some people, but I
suggest you withhold judgement or criticism. Perhaps your illness
has aroused fears they could not face.

You are the patient

Well-meaning relations, friends and workmates are likely to step forward with offers of help, causing your spouse, children or your parents to resent these intrusions into their lives. You yourself may feel
that your disease is 'family business' and of no concern to anyone else.
I believe it is essential for you to discuss this with your family and for

you, not *them*, to make the important decisions about who you would like to see, and when and how often they should visit. It's up to you to set your own agenda, and is an essential step towards regaining control of your life. Talking to others may be the last thing you want to do as you try to gather your thoughts, make sense of what has happened, decide whether your situation is a crisis, tragedy, or challenge.

In one way or another, everyone in your life will be affected by what has happened, but you shouldn't ignore your needs in order to protect those around you; they need to remember who is the patient so they don't isolate you as they try to come to terms with their fears, or start to prepare for a future without you.

It can be extremely difficult to depend on others if they were once dependent on you. You may feel that you have no right to ask for help, that you are 'using' them, or that they have enough worries of their own. You may have to learn something about graciously accepting the help of others and not denying them the opportunity to feel wanted. Asking them for help can make them feel as if they have something to contribute and so increase their sense of worth.

It is not unusual for those who are dependent on you to ask, 'What will happen to me?' The only way through this crisis is to talk about it, not pretend it is an issue that will go away or can be attended to later. One of the ironies of the situation is that in comforting your family and friends, you can empower yourself – and you need as much empowerment as possible – but remember, there's a fine line between providing reassurance and becoming a bereavement counsellor.

Also remember, you are not dead until you die. Some people think that once they have cancer, they have no future and surrender all their obligations and responsibilities. The problem with this is that you give up control at a time when, in order to survive, you need it most. It's also possible that you'll live for years or decades after your diagnosis, so your actions could add an unnecessary load to your family's already heavy burden.

The importance of speaking up

There may be issues you and your family members are reluctant to discuss with each other, creating an impasse. Your wife, for example, may be concerned about your will but is afraid to mention the subject for fear you will regard her question as an indication that she does not believe you will recover; you may not want to talk about it for fear of tempting Fate. You may wish to discuss your fears but are afraid you will only be adding to theirs; they may wish to talk about what they believe to be your impending death, but are fearful this will add to your distress as well as theirs.

If you hide your fears in order to protect the feelings of those nearest and dearest to you, you may effectively cut off any possibility of communication, and so intensify your own sense of abandonment. In this scenario, everyone loses out. It's hard enough to deal with your disease, but even harder if everyone feels unhappy and isolated. If the effort required to suppress your feelings leaves you drained of vital energy, you could impede your recovery. You laugh when you're happy, so why hold back the tears if you're sad? Your psychological well-being depends on everyone being able to express their feelings. There never was a more important time than now to honour them. It's normal. It's healing.

Use your spouse, family and friends as sounding-boards to discuss what you know. Their opinions may help you to make better decisions for yourself, but it is inappropriate for them to urge you to undergo treatment against your will and is bound to add one more log to the burden you feel you're already struggling to carry.

These are issues few families ever talk about but it is important that you do, and there are some real therapeutic benefits as well. As Elisabeth Kübler-Ross points out, research has shown that the key reason why so many widows and widowers visit their doctors and attend clinics with a whole range of somatic symptoms is because they failed to deal with their grief and their guilt *while their spouse was still alive*.[1]

The only way to resolve this problem and avoid the possibility of isolation is for everyone to share their feelings, and share the emotional burden you are all carrying. The added benefit of this is that when people can talk about their feelings it allows them to feel sorry for themselves – a necessary and natural response at a time when they are feeling guilty that they aren't only feeling sorry for you.

Ground rules

To help you maintain your autonomy, particularly in hospital, you need to lay down some ground rules with your family, friends, doctor and other health professionals.

The cardinal rule is that you should always be in control. Never let anyone make decisions for you – unless you really want them to. Your spouse and friends may be well-meaning in their efforts to take over all your responsibilities and make all your decisions for you, but in so doing they may leave you with nothing to do but wait for their next move. In such a state of passivity and resignation, you may find it impossible to dig yourself out of your fox-hole and try to regain control of your life. This is *your* battle, but you cannot fight it if you take orders from your army of supporters.

The responses of your family and friends can be a cause of great confusion and distress, more so if they wear long, mournful looks. Despite the advances in treatments, they may believe a cancer diagnosis is a sentence of death and so, unaware that they are being driven by their own fears and anxieties, urge you to be what they need you to be in order to cheer *themselves* up with catch-cries of 'Be positive! You'll be up and about before you know it'.

They may make excuses to stay away to avoid being reminded of their own mortality or of getting your disease, or because they feel so helpless at their inability to relieve your suffering or pain. If these people are important to you and their absence upsets you, tell them you would be pleased to see them when they are ready.

Family and other visitors may prattle on about matters of no interest to you, without any sensitivity as to your state of mind, and with little regard for your need to rest and consolidate your thoughts – until they feel they have done their duty, by which time you may be too exhausted to ask them to leave. Others may attempt to extract meaning from your condition even as they struggle to support and console you. They may be ignorant of your belief system or how you plan to cope, and may utter thoughtless or inappropriate statements such as 'It's God's will' or 'Don't worry, it's in God's hands'. They may feel as if they have said the right thing, but it could cause terror in your mind if, for example, you feel that what has happened to you is some form of divine retribution because you stopped going to church 20 years ago. Religious beliefs can be a source of great consolation, but not if you're an atheist, and not if you hold a different faith from those evangelical rescuers who urge you to 'speak in tongues or else you won't get better,' or tell you, 'All you have to do is confess your sins and God will heal you.'

If you feel you are losing control and would rather not listen to things that don't interest you, reclaim control by setting your own agenda up front. If there is something you want to share or discuss, tell them what *you* want to talk about. You're not being rude, you're being honest. You will, however, almost certainly drive people away if you use emotional blackmail or even direct threats such as, 'You didn't visit me yesterday. I had such a bad day.' Or, 'I feel so much better when I see you. It's a pity you don't visit more often.'

Your recovery depends, to a large extent, on ensuring you do everything at your own pace. This can be difficult if you have fixed appointments for treatments or tests, and even harder if you're in hospital and find yourself subjected to a rigid schedule of bed changes, meals, and physical examinations by doctors and nurses. This is not a time for you to be concerned with social correctness or feel obliged, for example, to see someone who has travelled a great distance to see you. You have the right to claim your own space if you don't feel up to the occasion, or if you feel depressed after a certain person has visited you. Ask your spouse, partner, friend, or the ward sister to filter all telephone calls, and check with you beforehand if you wish to see or avoid a particular visitor. Can't think of a suitable excuse? Ask those who are caring for you to tell your unwanted guests that you're sleeping.

What your carers should know

People who suddenly find themselves caring for someone with cancer react in various ways. Some people feel they have to be rescuers, and relish their role; others feel that they have had a load of added responsibilities dumped upon them, and become resentful. Some people feel that it is their duty to take care of their spouse, parent or child, without outside help; others marshal everyone within telephone reach to be at their beck and call. All these issues need to be addressed, particularly if recovery time is likely to last for weeks or months – and especially if recovery appears uncertain. The strain can be overwhelming, but there are ways to relieve this.

The person in your care is not dead until he or she dies. It is not uncommon for families to regard someone with cancer as having no future and so, in preparation for that time, relieve them of all obligations and responsibilities while they are still alive. If you do this, you not only deprive your family of that person's contribution to the family, but make the patient feel unwanted, isolated and lonely. Their will to live could be severely diminished by your actions.

The first and vital rule is that you should never make decisions for the person in your care – unless she asks you or is incapable of looking after herself. Take care – don't take over. You may be well-meaning in your efforts to assume all responsibilities and make all decisions for her, but in so doing you may leave her with nothing to do but wait for your next move. In such a state of reliance, she may find it impossible to regain control of her life.

It is important that you bear in mind that despite her possibly changed appearance and apparent lack of interest in matters that once seemed so important, she is still a person with human fears, needs and expectations. If you want to show you care, listen to her, acknowledge her feelings, and be careful you don't project your fears onto her even though you may feel that she is emotionally stronger than you. If you say, 'Don't worry, it's nothing,' or 'C'mon! It's not all that bad,' in an effort to cheer her up, to them it may seem as if her feelings count for nothing. She will feel even more isolated if you denigrate her views of her disease and her treatment program. She needs your endorsement, not your disregard or devaluation. One of the cruellest forms of abuse is to disregard someone else's feelings. Even if you have been through a similar situation, you cannot use your experience as a yardstick. Everyone is entitled to their individual feelings.

You convey your disregard for someone's feelings when you say, 'Oh, it's nothing,' or if you say, 'Don't be silly. You're imagining things'. Your criticism is out of place. The way to someone's heart is not to ignore it, but to listen to its beat.

Ask the person in your care to appoint someone as spokesperson or advocate, get the doctor to explain to the spokesperson as much about her illness and treatment as possible, and allow her to delegate responsibilities around the home. This is important for a number of reasons. Concerned family and friends tend to keep asking the same questions, and she will tire herself out having to answer them repeatedly. Everyone needs breathing space, so draw up a timetable for family members and friends who wish to become active participants in the care roster. In a time of chaos, the discipline of a timetable can restore order, allow everyone to commit themselves to times when they want to help, and alleviate their anxieties about the person who needs care in their absence.

If she lives on her own, or has other reasons for not asking family and friends to help, check the Resource Guide at the back of this book, and suggest she joins a support group. Join yourself, especially if you're the sole caregiver – there aren't many people who can cope on their own, without any help or anyone to talk to.

Nothing stays the same

When someone you love and care about has been injured or diagnosed with an illness serious enough for them to be in hospital, your natural response will be one of concern for yourself as well as them. Your husband, for example, may be off work for some time, so your anxiety for him is reflected when you say, 'I don't know how Bob's going to manage just sitting around all day. He was always such an active person.' If you find yourself saying something like, 'How am I going to cope with Bob sitting around all day?' you reflect your own fears.

It's not uncommon for the patient to end up comforting you, so that the line between who is the patient and who is the carer becomes somewhat blurred. This can work to your mutual advantage if each of you gains strength from one another. You are, however, bound to be angry and resentful if the patient uses his or her condition to manipulate you, is petulant and demanding, insists on special treatment, or adopts passive-aggressive behaviour. How to manage change is, perhaps, the most difficult challenge we all face. If, however, you accept that the process is one of transformation and that nothing stays the same, your ability to cope will be greatly enhanced.

So what can you do when he or she comes home? How can you make the transition less painful?

Things to guard against

- You, your family – even doctors – need to guard against dismissing complaints about lesser symptoms as trivial. This indifferent attitude can arise out of the belief that beside cancer nothing else is worth bothering about. You need to know that having a life-threatening disease is no guarantee that a person won't suffer from anything else. As a result of their compromised immune system, people who have had cancer are often more prone to diseases, including other cancers.

- Be prepared to acknowledge that things are rarely the same after a cancer diagnosis. You may hope, and even believe, that restoring the status quo is helpful, but this seldom happens.

- You need to guard against the isolating influence of changed perceptions of each other. For example, the person in your care may withdraw because he feels that his sense of worth has been devalued or that, with no future in common with those around them, he has nothing more to share. At the same time, you, your family and friends may stop sharing your thoughts and spend less of your time with him because you feel you have no future in common with someone who is sick or dying. People with cancer are often treated as if they were dying and so are isolated at a time when they are battling to stay alive.

- Beware of false expectations. You may be shocked to find that your perception that people with cancer become emaciated is wrong. I recall how isolated I felt when people said, 'You don't look like someone who is dying,' or, 'You don't look sick; why don't you go back to work?'

- Changed priorities often result in changed relationships: good marriages tend to become better, bad ones tend to become worse; children who once seemed preoccupied with their own instant gratification tend to become kind and caring, others, unable to cope, become angry and withdrawn.

- It is important that you support any event that helps you all feel better. This may involve encouraging visits from people who are vital and caring, and discouraging – perhaps even stopping altogether – visits from those who weep constantly or look like undertakers. It may also mean joining a support group on your own, or with your spouse/partner; arranging for help from a nursing service or a hospice; asking your doctor to visit more often.

☞ You may believe that the person will die or be committed to an institution, so you may experience the same feelings as if he had already died or gone away. There is a real danger here in that you behave in front of him as if he had already died.

At a time when he needs more contact to ease his suffering, any withdrawal is bound to add to his sense of isolation and depression – and even hinder his possible recovery. If he feels as if no one cares about him, why should he care about himself?

☞ Many people withdraw in order, they believe, to protect their family and friends from witnessing their suffering. Such stoic behaviour not only serves no useful purpose, it usually alienates the very people they wish to protect and exacerbates their grief.

☞ In every situation where we are compelled to deal with the pain and suffering of others, we need to address our own fears and anxieties or else we cannot truthfully attend to theirs. All too often we see in them our own vulnerabilities and frailties.

Nothing will be achieved by blaming them for actions and behaviour you feel may have contributed to their disease or injury. You also run the risk of showing anger instead of compassion if you make it clear you feel they aren't trying hard enough or if, in your opinion, they are not being assertive or active enough.

☞ Your choice of words can have the opposite effect to the one you intend if you say, 'I know just how you feel.' This remark may reflect your desire to show empathy, but it will surely reveal your utter lack of it. Unless you have had cancer or come close to death, you *can never* know what it's like – and even if you have, your reaction could be quite different from theirs.

☞ You should try to avoid burdening the person in your care with guilt by, for example, saying 'Don't die,' or 'How will we manage without you?' or 'When do you plan to return to work? Our debts are mounting.' If he is unable to return to work in the foreseeable future, if at all, what can he do?

It can be a tough time all round, and there is no magic formula that will help everyone cope with all the changes. You can work towards a resolution of your problems by recognising and being sensitive to each other's needs, and by remembering the wisdom of the adage: 'A joy shared is doubled, a sorrow shared is halved.'

How to communicate with someone who has cancer

Many people probably don't know how to communicate with someone who has cancer. They tend to assume that if they don't bring up the subject, the person with cancer won't either, sparing everyone the embarrassment of facing reality.

They may avoid using the word 'cancer', and even refer to it as 'you-know-what'. When they do discuss the illness, they may lower their voices when conversation comes to 'the word' as if they'll catch it by saying it aloud. You may be one of those who are uncertain as to whether your approach will be construed as too forward or too patronising, so you hold back and say nothing. If you do, the person who is ill may be wondering, 'What do they know that I don't?' Others' refusal to discuss or even mention the issue that is on everyone's mind can make the person with cancer feel quite isolated.

In people with cancer, the fear of death and overwhelming sense of impending loss is surpassed only by the fear that you and others will see that they are afraid and will abandon them; often they create a distance between themselves and others as a way of coping. They may also be concerned about how others will manage without them, and agonise that they are a burden on their families. Their feelings will fluctuate, so you may be disconcerted by different moods and changed behaviour (see previous chapter). You should not take these responses personally. The patient may not understand his own responses. Unless he is unaware of what is going on, do your best to include him in all discussions and decisions about his care and well-being. Patients with cancer want greater closeness from family and friends, not patronising and insensitive comments and actions.

People with a life-threatening disease instinctively have a good idea of whether they are going to live or die, so respect their privacy and their silence. They need the opportunity to make contact in their own time, on their terms. They want to be treated with consideration, and they want to be heard.

Under normal circumstances, it can often be difficult to get people to listen to you, but when you are seriously ill, it can be even harder, as those around seem to be doing all the talking. Now is the time to develop the art of listening. Don't dominate. Let the patient set the agenda and respond accordingly – and don't make assumptions about how he feels or what he wants. Take your cue from him. Find out what he wants to talk about, and if he doesn't want to talk, try touch. Words are seldom helpful if someone is frightened or aware they are going to die. Simply being present or holding hands, hugging, stroking or kissing can relieve his anxieties, discomfort or pain.

Pity is the worst emotion you can express as it will reveal your fear; rather, show compassion and reveal the extent of your love. You and the person you've come to visit may not get another chance to talk about things that have been left unsaid or issues that have not been resolved. Don't let the opportunity pass by either of you, but if the patient doesn't want to discuss the matter, don't force it.

Be prepared to laugh with him, even cry with him, but don't be overly solicitous. Unnatural passivity and solemnity can be unpleasant, and it can make you seem patronising. Long mournful looks should be banned. If you're still not sure how to be the best visitor you can be, ask yourself, 'How would I like to be treated if I were facing a life-threatening disease?' Let your honest answer be your guide.

WHAT NOT TO SAY
Trip over your shoe-laces, and you can always do them up again; trip over your tongue and you may regret it. These examples should give you an idea of what to avoid.

☞ 'Hello, old son! What are you doing here? On holiday again? Ha-ha-ha-ha!'

☞ 'Hello, Sam. Gee you look well. Taking a busman's holiday, are we? Well, don't worry! You'll be out of here before you know it.'

☞ 'Hello, Alice dear. We can't stay long; we're on our way to the movies, but we thought we'd just pop in for a minute to say hello.'

☞ 'Well, well, well! What have we got here, then? Harold not giving you enough TLC, huh?'

☞ 'I don't know how you did it, mate, but you sure picked the ward with the best-looking nurses!'

☞ 'Everything will be OK as long as you're positive.'

☞ 'Everything happens for the best.'

WHAT NOT TO DO

☞ Don't walk over to the person in the bed opposite and start talking to them.

☞ Don't sit down, pick up the newspaper and start reading.

☞ Don't watch the television above the bed.

☞ Don't start talking about what you have been doing since you last saw each other – unless you're asked.

☞ Don't lean forward and repeat all the latest rumours you've heard – unless you're asked.

☞ Don't tell them what they should have done to avoid getting ill.

☞ Don't read the chart at the foot of their bed as if you were a doctor, and nod your head knowingly.

☞ Don't tell stories about someone who had a bad experience with a doctor or hospital.

CHECKLIST OF DOS AND DON'TS FOR VISITORS

☞ Don't overstay your welcome. People with cancer get tired, but out of politeness may not ask you to leave. Give yourself a fixed time, then leave.

☞ Don't rush in and rush out. At the best of times, this would make someone feel unwanted. Be prepared to spend some time.

☞ Make several shorter visits rather than occasional over-long ones.

☞ Don't keep looking at your watch.

☞ Try to maintain eye contact, and keep your eyes at the same level. Don't keep looking away; show you're interested.

- Don't talk about your future with someone who may not have one.
- Ask her if she wants to talk, and if she does, make sure you listen. If she doesn't, put out your hand; touch is the most reassuring of the senses.
- If you can't hear her properly, don't pretend you can; ask her to repeat what she said.
- Don't change the subject, and don't keep interrupting.
- If you don't know what to say, tell her you don't know what to say.
- Don't give advice unless you're asked for it.
- Don't sit around gloomily as if you are at a funeral.
- Don't go on and on about a subject unless asked to. You may be excited about the football results – he couldn't care less.
- Don't expect to be entertained by the person you are visiting.
- Check with the family or the hospital first before giving the person you are visiting a drink, something to eat, or some medication you think will help them recover.[2]

What everyone should know about getting better

Most people assume that once you have cancer you are going to die, and they start to prepare themselves for the event. What they find much harder to deal with is your recovery. There can even be some resentment – after having resigned themselves to what they considered was your inevitable fate, now they have to readjust to your presence rather than your absence.

Facing your own recovery can be equally, if not more, daunting. Most people believe they will be excited when their treatment has stopped and they return home to their family and previous job or pastime. What they usually find is that they are depressed and cannot understand why.

It is normal to feel depressed at the prospect of an unplanned and open field of life before you if your life was centred around your treatment, from one visit after another to your doctor or clinic, being attended to 24 hours a day, and taking life 'one day at a time'. Life will feel different when you discover there isn't another appointment to keep, when the familiar faces of those who visited and nursed you have all gone, and you find it hard to picture them. Your depression may become even more acute if you fear your disease may recur and wonder what to do about it in the meantime.

It is not uncommon for those who cared for you to find they are also now at a loss as to what to do, and how to live life in the face of *their* fear that your disease will recur. They may not only find it hard to lead a normal life again – like you, they may not want to. A cancer scare tends to change everyone's priorities, and alter their views on the meaning of life. Keeping the lines of communication open throughout this trying time can help all of you reach depths of understanding of each other – and yourself – you may not otherwise have been able to achieve. You may also find it helpful to keep the following points in mind:

☞ Learn what you can about the problem. The antidote to fear and helplessness is knowledge.
☞ Talk about it. Communication is the antidote to isolation. Say what you expect of each other.
☞ Set realistic goals you can both manage.
☞ Agree on who has control of what, when, and how.
☞ Ask for help. Carers and patients alike all need 'time out'.
☞ Listen to each other. As in music, the pauses between the notes are often more meaningful than the notes themselves.

The importance of a cancer support group

People with cancer and their families often find themselves alienated from their former roles and positions in society. To help them make sense of their situation, they seek others who have had similar experiences, and often form a special bonding with them. A cancer support group is a group of people just like you, meeting regularly to talk about common issues, and providing emotional as well as physical support to each other. Based on the collective experiences of its members, it can provide you with much useful information, such as where to go for a second opinion, to whom and where to go for counselling, and where you can obtain specific information about your disease.

Some people resist joining support groups, especially if they live in a small town where everyone knows everyone else. You may be concerned that people will gossip so you won't be able to express yourself honestly. It has been my experience that people in support groups are very respectful towards, and protective of, each other. There is ample evidence to show that you can improve your chances of survival by reaching out and joining a cancer support group. A study conducted in the USA found a link between social isolation and mortality; that people who attend support groups feel better *and live longer*.[3] Your family can be your bulwark against depression, loneliness and fear; and provide you with support in managing those things you now find hard or impossible to do, but a support group can provide you – and your family – with that extra help to get you through. It can be vital if you are single or living on your own, and have no friends or family.

A bit further down the track, a support group can be invaluable in informing you about relaxation and diet, how to get to and from treatments, what local community services are available to meet your specific needs, how to deal with practical problems following, for example, a colostomy or ileostomy, and how to cope with relationships, existing and future. Solving specific problems is often more easily achieved in a group of like-minded people – and people who join cancer, heart and AIDS support groups are very focused on trying to solve their problems.

Perhaps the most useful contribution of a group is that it provides you with the best opportunity to meet and talk to others who, like yourself, have come face-to-face with a life-threatening disease. In such a unique environment a fellowship is created, in which there are no distinctions of age, sex, social status or economic class. In a support group everyone is equal – as we all are in the face of suffering and death. This is significant. When people are asked to list the main benefits of attending a support group, the phrase 'freedom to speak freely' usually tops the list; these people know how important it is to be able to keep re-telling their story, and the therapeutic value of this cannot be overemphasised. Thoughts that are unexpressed race round and round in your head, go nowhere, and cause great confusion and distress. Talking it out can calm the commotion in your mind, help you come to terms with your condition, allow you to see yourself and your disease from different perspectives, and help you bring your body's own healing powers into play.

People with cancer often think they are going crazy, and keep up a front to hide their fears and wild imaginings from their family, friends and doctors. Attending a support group will quickly help you realise that your feelings are normal. For example, you may be afraid of pain or that your cancer will recur, and so you conjure up images of yourself suffering or wasting away. Constrained by your desire to protect your family, you may be compelled to act differently from the way you feel. In a group, you can share feelings you're not used to sharing with your family, and say things you would not otherwise say. Learning how to express yourself in a group will make it easier for you to do so at home.

To an outsider, the idea of joining a cancer support group may conjure up images of doom and gloom, but far from it! As most people soon discover, attending a support group makes you feel better and safer through a mutual giving and receiving of feelings. It's agreeable to find and get to know other people who are supportive and care about you.

With few exceptions, most people find a support group helps them regain a sense of hope. Only other people who have been through the same experience as you can provide you with this unique source of inspiration and support; only another cancer patient can truly understand what you are going through. As one member of a breast cancer support group once said, 'A support group lets us talk like sisters.' Being able to express your feelings reduces your sense of isolation, introduces a sense of community. In a group, you do not have to face your fears alone.

People in groups learn to give themselves, rather than giving things or money. In times of high anxiety, moral support is more highly valued than either physical or financial support.

It's not uncommon to find that your experience sets you apart, and that long-established relationships no longer satisfy you as you find you have less in common. A support group can not only introduce you to a network of new and interesting friends, it can provide you with a safe place in which you can be yourself, and explore new ways to understand yourself. Support groups can provide the love people often find lacking in their lives. This is as true for single and widowed people as it is for those with families.

A support group can also provide your husband, wife, partner, or other caregivers with the opportunity to make contact with other people away from your hospital or home environment. The fellowship these groups generate can do much to alleviate *their* sense of isolation as they care for you. Now they can always ask someone from the group to keep you company while they get time on their own or to see and talk to someone else, take in a movie, indulge in some 'shop' therapy, visit the hairdresser or dentist, or simply catch up on some well-earned sleep. Spending even a little time apart can provide everyone with much-needed breathing space.

Most support groups deal with general issues, some deal with specifics such as laryngectomy, ostomy, prostate, and breast cancer. There are many other resources you can draw on for support, so consult the Resource Guide at the back of this book. Help is always close at hand.

If you find yourself in a support group where the quality of leadership and the nature of the other participants do not inspire you, where you find yourself at variance with the thinking of the group, or where listening to ongoing tales of suffering distresses you, shop around, preferably for another group. Self-help groups can be self-righteous and highly critical of other groups, doctors and other health professionals. Some of the ideas supported by these groups present real risks, as in the case of Linda, following her diagnosis of breast cancer.

Linda attended a group where she was persuaded that all her problems, including her cancer, were caused by the traumas she had suffered during her childhood. Under normal clinical conditions, dealing with such issues is a drawn-out process, requiring great skill and intense emotional support on the part of the therapist. Linda received none of these, was made to feel guilty that she had not addressed these issues and, when she asked for ongoing help, was told it was up to her to sort out her life. Left to her own devices, Linda suffered such distress she required psychiatric intervention.

Be wary. Find a support group in which

☞ control of the group remains in the hands of the members;

☞ medical or psychiatric advice is not given by other members, but by doctors;

- your individual way of coping with your disease is respected;
- your cultural, religious and social values are respected;
- access to and information about your disease and its treatments, counselling, hospice, palliative care and local community services are provided.

The support group that best supports you is also the one that draws on outside resources. For example, many groups invite guest speakers to talk on a range of issues: an oncologist to talk about treating side effects, a beautician to talk about hair aids and make-up, a dietician to advise on a balanced, nourishing diet, a counsellor or psychologist to help deal with emotional issues. A support group that doesn't support you is not worth joining.

Part Four

making sense

of it all

twelve

restoring the balance
in your life

Your prayer must be that you have a sound mind
in a sound body; Pray for a bold spirit,
free from all dread of death.'

JUVENAL

The message of cancer

In Western societies, good health is taken for granted; ill health is associated with bad habits or bad luck. Many caregivers, including doctors, consider ill health a sign of weakness, and so adopt a paternalistic approach towards people when they are ill, treating them as weak and helpless children, victims and objects of pity. A life-threatening disease is also an unwelcome reminder to everyone around you of the inevitable passing of life.

To get through the eye of the storm, you need to remind yourself that good health cannot be taken for granted, and that disease is an integral part of the human condition. A life-threatening or chronic disease can teach you about survival, and remind you that while you can often overcome disease, you cannot conquer death. It begs you not to abuse your good health, and demands you try to find balance in your life. It shows you that the opposite of fear is not fearlessness, but courage, and that the things that become important are the things that are important. It even reminds you that you may die before your parents or your children.

There will be times when it's hard to keep this perspective – times when your fears and anxieties overshadow your hopes and joys. This can happen even after you have recovered, when a visit to your doctor for a check-up or a drive past the hospital where you had your treatment reminds you of the more frightening times you endured and may even cause some of the physical symptoms you experienced during treatment to recur – fortunately these are usually milder, and pass fairly quickly.

It may be hard for you to imagine this right now, but further down the track – perhaps when you reach 5 or 10 AD (After Diagnosis) – you may remember, with a sigh of relief and a sense of gratefulness, how your life once seemed to be suspended by a thread, but is now more securely tethered.

Facing reality, living in the present

People deal with problems in their own way, some more successfully than others. You may take the view that the best way is to put your disease out of your mind, keep busy in order to distract yourself, and hope the problem will go away. You may find your disease and its treatments all too much to bear, pretend it's not your problem, and leave everything to your doctor and your family.

These coping strategies may provide you with temporary relief, but they are a retreat from reality. What happens when, alone with your thoughts, your anxieties refuse to go away? Worrying about a situation you feel powerless to influence saps your energy, destroys your will, and keeps you focused on the difficulties facing you rather than looking for ways to overcome them. Your response may be, 'What's the use?' – especially if the prognosis is grim, you feel there is no quality of life, or your advanced age tells you there is so little to look forward to, that you 'mark time' by reminiscing.

I cannot comment on your decision to adopt this approach if you are very old, as my experience of old people tends to be coloured by the way my father coped with his advancing age. Dad lived with me until he died aged 87, at home, of a last heart attack. The previous 23 years of his life were spent dealing with three heart attacks, high blood pressure and chronic arthritis. He constantly reminisced, and held everyone in thrall as he related his adventures and remarkable skirmishes with death through two world wars on two continents. He never worried about his health, believed worrying about what was going to happen was futile. He never lost hope he would endure – as he did – to see his grandchildren grow up and reach their various milestones.

I share his views. There can be no going forward when you are chained to the past, locked in by your fears, and bound by no hope. You stand little chance of coping with your cancer, even less of relieving your misery, if dwelling on the past and worrying about the future prevents you from living in the present. The most effective strategy is to confront the problem, act accordingly, and *let whatever happens in the future flow from your actions rather than your fears*. I know it isn't easy when you feel 'stressed out', but there is always more than one solution to a problem – and the only one that's right is the one that's right for you, not your spouse, partner, family or friends. Your life and theirs may run in tandem, but you can only live your own life. In *The Prophet*, Kahlil Gibran, poet and mystic, summed this up well:

> *And stand together yet not too near together:*
> *For the pillars of the temple stand part,*
> *And the oak tree and the cypress grow not in each other's shadow.*

The issue of stress

By definition, stress means any situation or condition that causes you hardship, disquiet and discomfort. It can take various forms: work-related pressures, relationship conflicts, financial burdens, the loss of a loved one, a diagnosis of cancer.

Humans have survived for millennia thanks mainly to our built-in 'fight-or-flight' mechanism. Confronted by danger, we need extra energy in order to fight off our attacker, or to escape. Our heart rate and breathing increase, and our bodies undergo changes to meet the sudden demand for energy. In the modern world, where we have a deadline to meet, a speech to make or a match to win, we can use the increased energy – properly channelled – to give us the winning edge. However, in situations where we have no one to fight and no-where to run, all that angry or fearful energy builds up. Our bodies react with heart palpitations, sweating, increased stomach acidity, stomach spasms, skeletal muscle spasms – and increased blood pressure. We begin to stew. Like a nuclear power plant that can't be cooled down, and without an outlet for all that energy, we start our own meltdown. The chain reaction can be disastrous. Over time, instead of getting better, we get worse. Our immune system takes a battering.

Fear of the unknown causes the same responses and lowers our tolerance to pain and discomfort. Although everyone has a different personality style, knowing what to expect and learning as much as you can about your condition prepares you for what lies ahead, and can help ease your anxiety. You can't turn the clock back and rectify the stressful situations which may have contributed to your disease, so it's your distress (your response) to your current situation with which you need to cope rather than the stress (the cause). Before describing the ways in which you can handle your distress, it is important you know how your responses affect you, and to understand that there is no difference between listening to the wisdom of your body or your mind.

The immune system and stress

The immune system was once considered autonomous and completely unaffected by any internal, regulatory mechanisms. It used to be thought that whatever memory it had was limited to recognising foreign bodies (germs and viruses) it had previously encountered and destroyed.

It was later discovered that our first line of defence against foreign organisms is orchestrated by our innate immunity in the form of one group of white cells called leukocytes, and that there is a second line of defence in another group of white cells called lymphocytes. Lymphocytes gives us adaptive immunity. They adapt because they 'remember'. What makes them even more remarkable is that the lymphocytes in our blood have neuro-receptors on them – just as do those parts of the brain that affect emotion and stress.

What this means is that the immune system and the central nervous system interact, and that the immune system, far from being independent, can and *does* receive and send messages from and to the brain through hormones, chemical messenger molecules known as *neurotransmitters*, that move through our blood, and from cell to cell in our brain. Neurotransmitters, also known as neuropeptides, are secreted by the brain, the immune system and by nerve cells.

They transmit signals from one nerve to another nerve or cell structure to obtain a response, for example, a nerve impulse or a muscle contraction.

In this way, the central nervous system co-ordinates behavioural and immune responses during stressful situations. Physical stress and emotion activate the hypothalamus which, in turn, triggers the pituitary gland to releases a stress hormone, corticotropin-releasing hormone (or CRH), through the bloodstream to the adrenal glands, which lie above the kidneys. These glands, which are part of the body's hormone system, then release corticosteroids which perform two main functions: they arouse the body to fight or flee when faced with trouble, and they modulate the body's immune system. Anything that inhibits the continued release of CRH lowers our immune defences, and increases our susceptibility to diseases, inflammatory conditions such as rheumatoid arthritis, and behavioural syndromes such as depression, anxiety and anger.[1] Corticosteroids also affect gene expression, that is, the way cells communicate with each other; they tell cells when to grow or divide – and if a gene is expressed at the wrong time in a cell's life cycle, cancer can result.[2]

What's in your mind will find its way into your body

In everyday terms, this means that our thoughts and emotions are in direct communication with our immune system: what we think and what we feel – consciously or unconsciously – can raise or depress our hormone and immune levels.[3] Continued long-term lowering of these levels can eventually erode our health, give rise to a variety of diseases, including auto-immune disorders such as pernicious anaemia, lupus, myasthenia gravis, rheumatoid arthritis, heart disease and cancer.

What's in your mind will find its way into your body, and it happens every day in so many ways. For example, if you feel depressed, your shoulders sag, you get a headache, find you can't sleep. Or, if you get angry, your face goes red, you start to shake, your heart and breathing rates go up. Over many years, the effect of all the things that are 'eating you up' becomes cumulative. Our diseases become metaphors for our fears, resentments, lack of love, being misunderstood.

Remember, the word 'immune' comes from the Greek word for memory, the very attribute our immune system shares with our central nervous system. The good memory which is essential to the smooth working of the immune system means that your body also remembers your past bad experiences and the way you responded to them. If you can recognise this, you can look at your illness, not as a disease but as a message to change, to find out what it is about your life you need to alter so you can improve its quality and, perhaps, increase its length.

The immune system has a sophisticated memory system, but it cannot differentiate between the unintended and the intended input. It is like a computer: it will do what it is programmed to do, but it cannot think. When we use words that reflect our state of mind, they imprint themselves on our bodies:

'I can't stand this any more.'

'I can't take any more of this.'

'I've had enough!'

'This is all too much for me.'

'I wish I were dead.'

You may have spent your life committing suicide by default when, in the face of continuing disappointments, unresolved issues at home or at work and your apparent inability to do anything right, you kept wishing you were dead, somewhere else, any convenient way of relieving your anguish.

Many of the people I have counselled for cancer and other life-threatening illnesses have told me how, at various stressful times, they had wished to die. In particular, some felt as if they had never got what they wanted, others that they had lived lives of unfulfilled love. They felt, and finally discovered, to their dismay, that disease can provide a socially acceptable form of suicide as it did for Jack, whose story I described in the previous chapter. He desperately wanted a way out of his marital problems, kept putting off the inevitable, used to say, 'If I don't walk out of here, they'll carry me out.' Eventually diagnosed with leukemia, he realised that his body-mind had taken him literally, so he fought back and survived.

Our immune system is not only affected by our thoughts, words, and external threats, but by our habits: not getting enough sleep, not eating enough, consuming tobacco, alcohol, caffeine, tranquillisers and other drugs. Ainslie Meares, renowned psychiatrist and author, summed this up concisely when he said, 'We are built into a pattern of life by the way we live.'[4]

In spite of the mounting evidence of the mind–body connection, many doctors still believe that your genes are solely to blame for causing cancer, and that psychosomatic medicine should be limited to treating hypochondriacs. The view that 'it's all in your mind' ignores the mounting evidence that what's in your mind and in your body are intimately linked by neurotransmitters. Admittedly, some cancers are inherited, such as retinoblastoma, familial polyposis and multiple endocrine neoplasia; others occur in people who are more at risk, such as daughters of women with breast cancer and first-degree relatives of individuals with lung cancer, especially if they smoke cigarettes.[5] As I said earlier, there is nothing you can do about your parents; other cancers are caused by genes that mutate after birth as a result of damage by radiation, smoking, alcohol. Others arise from several causes – perhaps a mixture of genetic predisposition, lifestyle, the environment, and chance. The contribution of mind–body interactions cannot be discounted. We need to keep reminding ourselves of some basic truths, perhaps best expressed in the words of Sai Baba, who said, 'One's anger is one's greatest enemy, and one's calmness is one's protection. One's joy is one's heaven, and one's sorrow is one's hell'.

Stress and cancer

In his book, *On Being Human*, anthropologist Ashley Montagu reminds us that 'each cell depends for its proper functioning upon the interaction with it of every other cell of the organism.'[6] In the same way as the survival of a species depends on the mutual co-operation of its members in warding off attack, so a threat to one cell represents a threat to all cells, and ultimately to the survival of the entire bodymind.

Maintaining mutual co-operation so the body can survive means all cells need to be in uninterrupted communication with each other, reproduce only when signalled to do so by other cells, and maintain their rightful place in the scheme of things. When everything is in order, and the immune system and the central nervous system are in harmony, the body is said to be in steady state called *homeostasis*. But this delicate balance is continually under threat from germs, viruses, the environment in which we live and the way we respond to stressful situations, some present, others long gone but still unresolved. There is a popular view that cancer originates from a stressful event that occurred in the previous eighteen months, but generalising in this way is wrong. There are over 100 different forms of cancer, and for one to grow to the size of a pea can take from six months to 20 years or more; it all depends on the type of cancer – some cancers grow slowly, some grow rapidly. The length of time between onset and diagnosis is often so long that the primary cause can't always be identified, although, as I will discuss in the following chapter, it is my belief that a predisposition towards many cancers can be traced back to traumatic events in childhood.

Just as it takes only one straw to break a camel's back, so the 'trigger' that finally upsets our bodymind's natural balance and stimulates cancer's unrestrained and rampant cell growth can be anything from smoking to bereavement, sunbathing to poor diet. In most instances, the interval between the cause and the effect is so great we fail to locate the cause of our disease, blaming it on something or someone else, preferably something that occurred more recently.

Where there *is* a clear connection, it is foolish to avoid doing something about the 'trigger'. For example, if you used to smoke and have been treated successfully for lung cancer, it is absurd to take up smoking again; if you have unresolved issues, you have to attend to them. To do so effectively, you will need to stiffen your resolve and show you are not afraid; discover that life is to be celebrated, death not to be feared. You probably can't change the stressful situations around you, but you can change your attitude, your perspective and your priorities. The greatest courage you can show is to face reality head-on and allow yourself to be seen for who you really are – and to accept this as one of the ultimate truths.

So how can you restore order? Can the immune system learn new tricks, forget old patterns? Can you enhance your immune function?

Stress and distress

When we say we're 'stressed out', or that our 'stress levels are too high', what we really mean is that we're in pain, are having problems or conflicts that are making us *distressed*. Distress is our reaction to stress: anger, worry, fear, depression. Distress is our response to any situation over which we feel we have little or no control. Your distress levels could be so high they're affecting your response to your treatment, slowing down your recovery, and diminishing the quality of your life. You may be unusually intolerant of those around you or indifferent to what happens next. You may find difficulty in making decisions or experience memory problems.

Distress can reveal itself in various other ways – when we're feeling panicky, uneasy, angry, powerless, depressed, grief-stricken, isolated, trapped. At a physical level, distress is revealed through symptoms such as fatigue, heart palpitations, confusion, tightness of chest, sweaty, dry mouth, muscle tensions, insomnia, irritability, loss of sex drive, decreased appetite. You know you are distressed when you think thoughts such as, 'I can't breathe, I can't do it, I'm trapped, I'm not going to get out of here, I can't manage alone, no one will help.'

Clearly, if your response to stressful situations is always the same, you reinforce the effects and condition your bodymind to repeat old patterns. Behaviour that is not rewarded does not continue. If you train yourself to respond differently, you can break the cycle. What your bodymind learned through past experience, you now have to teach it to unlearn. There is no quick solution, but if you persevere you can succeed.

Facing cancer can challenge even the most optimistic person, but if you can try to see your cancer as a 'fight or flight' situation, you can use the energy it gives you to keep going, to try to understand more about it (the stress) and yourself (the distressed), so you won't see yourself as helpless or dependent, and give up. If you adopt the 'flight' response, you will discover that the best place to run is not to a place, since there is nowhere to hide, but to a space you create when you meditate or do nothing; if you adopt the 'fight' response, you will discover it's not your cancer you have to fight (leave that to your cancer specialist), but your fears.

How to deal with distress

Instead of asking, 'How can I cope with my distress?' you need to ask, 'What specific problem or conflict is making me feel like this?'

Cancer and its treatments can cause depression which is often hard to distinguish from distress. Anti-depressants and stress management techniques only deal with symptom control, so pinning down the cause of your distress may require professional help from a psychiatrist or a counsellor. You need to be realistic about your condition, and give yourself time to deal with all your unresolved issues.

Relieving distress

You can combat your negative thoughts, feelings and physical responses by replacing them with positive ones. It takes practice, but you can do it. Beware you don't become a prisoner of positive thinking, believing that all you have to do is repeat positive affirmations continuously and your cancer will go away. Positive thinking without positive action is futile. Try these statements:

- If you say, 'I feel trapped', turn it around and say, 'I feel trapped at this moment, but there are still things I can do that can make me feel free.'
- If you keep saying, 'I'm so tired,' say instead 'I feel tired now – but I know I will feel better when I've taken a nap.'
- If you find pain makes you fearful, say to yourself, 'Yes, I am afraid of pain – but if I talk to my doctor I'm sure he'll give me something to get rid of it.'
- If you say, 'I look terrible', turn it around to 'Yes, I look terrible right now because I've had chemo – but my hair will grow back, I will look better.'
- If you say to yourself, 'I'm going to die', rather say, 'I know I'm going to die, eventually, but in the meantime I am going to get better.'

Remember, your immune system can't think, but it has a good memory. At all times try to use the word *when* instead of the word *if*. Talk to yourself. Say, again and again, 'I'm going to live,' instead of 'I'm going to die.' Say, again and again, 'I deserve to live,' instead of 'I wish I were dead.' As Ella Fitzgerald sang, 'Accentuate the positive, eliminate the negative.'

Whatever you do, don't blame yourself. Even if you were a heavy smoker and developed lung cancer, blaming yourself isn't going to help. You may feel as if you can't deal with your responses right now, but if you accept that, for the short term, you have lost control of the situation, say to yourself, 'Right now I have lost control, but I will regain it when I feel a little stronger.'

LISTEN TO YOUR BODYMIND

Our bodies and our thoughts talk to us. Most of the time, we tend to ignore them. I urge you to listen well, and to honour them. Your symptoms are as real as your fears. Accept them as normal responses to an abnormal situation and deal with them if you can. For example, if you feel tired, go to sleep, don't fight it off. If you feel afraid, ask yourself why. Listen to your bodymind; it's talking to you as clearly as your thoughts.

As I explained earlier, cells communicate with each other through neurotransmitters found in the brain and throughout the body. The language they speak ensures their and your survival by telling other cells what to do: make more of this protein and less of that, send more energy to the digestive system, and so on. You're the collection of all your cells, so there's no reason they can't talk to you. All you have to do is listen.

SLEEP

My late father used to say that when a dog is sick, it sleeps and doesn't eat. Over the years, doctors marvelled at the way he bounced back after each health setback and told me secretly they thought he had the answer, but not to quote them because 'it's not scientific'.

But they were wrong. Two separate reports in 1996 and 1997 have shown that going without sleep lowers lymphocyte levels, suppressing the immune system, and leaving your body more susceptible to infection. Don't fight off sleep. It's your body's way of saying, 'I want down-time. I can't keep going.' [7]

EXERCISE

Exercise can play a key role in restoring your bodymind's balance. Regular physical exercise can help reduce anxiety and mild depression, distract you from your misery, and raise your self-esteem.

Exercise stimulates the production of endorphins, the body's own morphine, to raise your pain threshold and help control any pain you may have. The most important benefit of exercise is that it is a series of movements over which you have complete control; any physical stress it may cause is under your command.

Physical exercise should not be tiring. To reap its full benefits, choose an exercise you like, and do it for no more than 20–30 minutes a day.

REACH OUT FOR HELP

You may think this is the right time to keep a stiff upper lip and show everyone around you how strong you are, how independent you can be.

If you had fallen into a raging torrent and someone reached out to save you, would you grab their hand and allow yourself to be saved, or would you say, 'No thanks, I'll tough this one out on my own'? It's OK to ask for help from your family, friends, your doctor and other caregivers.

There's a real downside to refusing help: apart from failing to relieve your distress, you may drive people away at a time when it is essential you maintain good social relationships. As Montagu reminds us in *On Being Human*, the more co-operative the group, the greater is the fitness for survival of all its members.

Reaching out for help also includes touching. Fear of contagion from cancer is so strong that many people pull away at a time when you most need the touch of their skin on yours. Touch is our first contact with reality. Throughout our lives, it provides our whole conception of what exists outside us. We can be deprived of all our senses, except touch, and still survive. Touch can stimulate or calm us; it is our first and most lasting association with love.

DO SOMETHING FOR YOURSELF

This is not the time for you to carry on as before or pretend you're in good health and can manage on your own. Your family and friends shouldn't expect you to do all the things you did for them before your diagnosis. You need to make sure you get enough rest, food and exercise. You need 'time out' to heal yourself.

Set aside as much time as you possibly can – anything from 20 minutes to an hour or more per day – to do the things you want to do *for yourself*. You will surely run out of time if you say you don't have the time. You can't afford to put your life on 'hold' if you want to give yourself a chance of fulfilling your dreams and enjoying the companionship of your family and friends – or whatever – for months or years to come.

'But my family needs me,' you say, or 'I have to think of my wife and children first,' or 'Who's going to pay the mortgage if I don't?'

If you regard yourself as the centre of your family's universe, or think you are indispensable, you not only have a misplaced sense of your own importance, you also have little faith in their ability to manage without you – which they will have to do anyway if you don't get better.

Maybe you should take time out to find out why you regard it as more important to satisfy everyone else's needs rather than your own at this point in your life – and do it now if you want to give yourself a chance of healing or to find the peace of mind that comes from accepting the inevitable.

KEEP A JOURNAL

Writing is no substitute for professional counselling, but it can help you express your feelings, your fears, your doubts and your hopes. Writing them out will help you focus on your day-to-day activities, and so help you keep track of how you are coping. As a bonus, it will help you gain new insights into yourself – especially if you regard what you write as private and for your eyes only.

It's hard to resolve problems while they're whirling around in your head. Putting pen to paper, finger to keyboard, helps you to see the issues that beset you in black and white. Seeing them in this detached way usually makes them more manageable, and it will keep you psychologically honest.

FORGIVENESS AND SELF-ESTEEM

Self-esteem is the value you place on yourself. No one can give it you. You raise your self-esteem when you do something for yourself because you think you're worth it. Your self-esteem can be reinforced when the choice you make in pursuing a particular course of action results in approval, success or recognition. With raised self-esteem, everything becomes possible. Moreover, people who think they're worth saving don't give up.

With lowered self-esteem, nothing seems possible, nothing worth the effort, and nothing will satisfy you. If, on top of this, you feel you are a victim of circumstances, you will feel depressed – and depression leads to even lower self-esteem, and suppresses your immune system.

You may think you're not worth saving for any number of reasons: because you believe cancer is nature's way of ensuring old age is not a burden on the young, or because you will become a liability to your family; perhaps you think you deserve your disease as punishment for some act or omission on your part, or you think you're a loser.

You can start by not blaming yourself for your disease, follow the guidelines in this and the following chapter; then re-read Chapter 10, and realise that the moment you lose interest in yourself, your life and your future, everyone else, of necessity, will lose interest in you.

You can recover your self-esteem if you forgive yourself as well as others. Forgiveness is the opposite of blame; you remove guilt and replace it with love, and leave the past behind, where it belongs.

Two Zen monks were on their way to a temple when they came upon a woman standing on the bank of a river. She saw them and immediately cried out, 'Please help me! I can't swim, and I have to cross the river to get to my village.'

One of the monks picked her up, and with his friend beside him, waded across the river to the opposite bank, where he put her down. She thanked him profusely and raced away.

The monks proceeded on their journey, and as they walked, the monk who had carried the woman wondered aloud, 'She shouldn't have been there alone. There are many bandits who would take her for ransom.' A little further on, he said, 'No father should let such a young woman travel unescorted.' Further on, he said, 'I wonder what she would have done if we had not passed her way?' By the time they reached their destination, his companion, tired of his continuing chatter, turned to him and said, 'Why are you still carrying her on your back?'

You can convert the passivity of guilt into constructive action by letting go of, and forgiving others for, any guilt and responsibility for what happened in the past, and by putting your pride in your pocket and asking for forgiveness from those you have wronged. It takes courage, but if you're not worth fighting for, who is?

There may be unresolved issues with people in your life, now and from the past. They may be people you don't have the courage to face, or perhaps they live too far away; maybe they have died. Writing them a long letter in which you express all your previously unspoken feelings – especially your anger and your hurt – can be a liberating experience, as it was for Rebecca, a woman I counselled.

Rebecca lived alone. Her husband had died several years earlier, and neither her daughter nor her grandchildren wanted anything to do with her. Rebecca had this daughter when she was sixteen and still at school. Her mother decided to bring up the little girl and sent Rebecca to live interstate. By the time she had completed high school, Rebecca had grown into a beautiful woman, attractive to many men. She enjoyed the good life. As the years went by, Rebecca's mother brainwashed her granddaughter about her 'useless' mother. Rebecca's daughter grew up, married and bore three children.

When Rebecca was diagnosed with lung cancer, she came to see me, her mental distress as palpable as her physical pain. She told me how she had tried, again and again, to meet her aged mother, daughter and grandchildren, but was always rebuffed. A cousin of hers kept her informed, showed her photographs of the family who would have nothing to do with her, but nothing could ease the pain of her loss. She was contrite, realised she had acted immaturely as a teenager, and was desperate to see her family.

'I never knew them before; now I'm going to die without ever seeing them,' she said. I suggested she write a letter to each of them, explaining how she felt, forgiving everyone for punishing her, and asking for forgiveness for what she had done. It took her several weeks to finish writing each of the letters, but she could not bring herself to post them. I suggested she burn them in the company of friends, champagne in hand. When I saw Rebecca a week later, her eyes were brighter, her step lighter. She was transformed, and felt she had expressed all her repressed hurts.

'What was, was,' she said. 'I'm glad I never actually posted those letters. They might have misunderstood me all over again.'

The story doesn't have a completely happy ending. Rebecca was diagnosed a few weeks later with an aortic aneurysm, and died without seeing her family, who didn't attend her funeral.

Burning the past may seem like a small ritual, but it can have a profound healing effect on you.

TAKE UP A HOBBY – PLAY

The mere mention of the word often draws responses such as, 'Who has the time to play?' and 'Hobbies are a waste of time – that's kids' stuff!'

The fact is, a hobby allows you to recapture the joy of play for that child within you who has never left you. It is important that you recognise him or her, because it is only by honouring all aspects of your self that you can regain the balance and control you have lost. If ever you needed permission to start playing again, your cancer just gave it to you.

Find something that lifts your spirits, revitalises your interest in life, and allows you to express the free spirit of the child within you. Your self-renewal may lie in music, gardening, knitting, painting, watching the waves break over and over again. Or what about buying a model train like the one that gave you so many hours of fun when you were a kid?

In play, you don't have to meet anyone else's expectations; you can give your imagination free rein, lose yourself so completely that nothing distresses you.

REARRANGE YOUR PRIORITIES

I have been asked by many people, 'Why is it necessary to complete my unfinished business?' and 'Why do I have to rearrange my priorities?'

It may not be necessary, but right now your world is in a mess. Everything is upside down and inside out. You may not have a soon-to-be fatal illness at this moment, but one thing is certain: death is always only a heartbeat away. Because of this fact, there are two questions life always puts to us:

1   If you are going to die in the relatively near future, what are you going to do with the remaining time you have left?

2   If you are going to die in the relatively later future, what are
     you going to do with the remaining time you have left?

It certainly won't do any harm to re-consider your priorities, and this
checklist should help you find out if you think you ought to change
them or not.

☞   Are you fearful of the future?
☞   Are you unsure of what the remaining time of your life holds
     in store for you?
☞   Are you afraid of death or the act of dying?
☞   Do you feel a pressing need to watch your children grow up?
☞   Are you unsure if you have provided for your children's
     financial and emotional future?
☞   Are you sure you have provided for your own future – in this
     life and, if you believe in it, in the next?
☞   Do you harbour any guilt for anything you've ever done?
☞   Do you have any regrets about anything you've done or did
     not do?
☞   Are there any wrongs you feel you may have suffered?
☞   Is there any wish you feel has not been fulfilled?
☞   Is there someone you have wronged or harmed whose
     forgiveness you would like?
☞   Is there someone you want to forgive for what they did to
     you?
☞   Have you opened your heart to those you closed it to?
☞   Have you made out a last will and a living will?

You may choose to continue doing what you did before your diagnosis, and if that is your choice, that is your right. However, I believe
that in the face of death anything is possible, that you now have, perhaps for the first time in your life, the opportunity (short of breaking
the law) to do what *you* want to do without the need for the approval
of anyone.

SPEAK UP
In the same way as putting pen to paper helps you express your inner
hurts and anxieties, so speaking up will relieve your distress.

Some people feel they're safer when they don't speak up, don't draw attention to themselves. This can often happen in a hospital where nursing care is not of the best, and where patients who say what they feel are marginalised, labelled as 'troublemakers' and not 'good patients'.

Speaking up will help you maintain your relationships with those around you as long as you express those feelings that belong to you and don't transfer them onto others. There is a difference between saying, 'I am unhappy at the treatment I am receiving,' and 'You treat me badly.' They may be temporarily upset at what you said, but will appreciate your honesty as soon as they realise you are not labelling them but claiming your own feelings.

There is no way you can release the pressure of unexpressed fears unless you speak up. Talking about how your cancer has affected your life, your role in the family, and your fears of dependency and abandonment will help you normalise your experience and put everything back into perspective. Make your needs known. Your distress will be greatly relieved if you know you will not be abandoned, will receive pain control when you need it, and will be treated with dignity.

And try saying, 'No.' Our fear of upsetting others is often greater than our fear of distressing ourselves. Assert your needs and you will find it easier to cope, define yourself to others, and say 'No!' to your cancer.

LOVE ALL – SERVE ALL

I understand what you're going through. I also know that as someone with cancer, you are qualified to comfort someone else with cancer.

You may feel you don't have the strength to help anyone except yourself, and right now that may be true. But if you've joined a support group, you'll know just how rewarding it can be – both for you and for everyone else – so as soon as you can, try to help someone else.

Helping others is a unique survival tool. Contrary to what most people have been led to believe, survival of the fittest does not mean that the weakest and the stupidest are selfishly exploited by the toughest and the shrewdest. History teaches us that fitness applies to the group rather than the individuals in it. Those tribes and nations that survive best have been those in which there is co-operation and love. It stands to reason, therefore, that each of us has a better chance of survival when we help and show love to one another.

There is a photograph on my desk of Sai Baba. The inscription on it is, 'Love all, serve all.' It is a constant reminder to me of a vow I made to myself when I was close to dying from cancer the first time (see Bargaining in Chapter 10).

Help others and you help yourself. If you can see yourself as a candle, you can be a source of light and warmth, and a beacon to others, but be careful they don't get so close they blow you out. You have to conserve some energy for yourself.

Do nothing

How often have you wished to do nothing, lie under a tree and look up at the sky, sit on a rock and watch the waves curl and break in front of you? In general, we are so busy working or attending to the needs of others, we fail to heed our bodymind's warning signals to slow down, and we get ill.

We share a vital need with all animals to rest, to do nothing except to be at one with nature. Instead, for many people, leisure time now means rushing from place to place, looking at nature through the lens of a camera, measuring their enjoyment by how much they can do in the time they have, afterwards saying, 'I need another holiday to recover.'

Listen to your inner self when it tells you to get in rhythm with nature – perhaps the best stress reliever of all. Provided you do it with intent, doing nothing isn't loafing – it's as important as doing something to relieve your distress, giving your bodymind time to heal.

Finding your space

The universe is a measureless, self-regulating organism – and that includes each and every one of us. Aristotle refers to the universe as a single organism in which each part grows and develops in its relationship to the whole in which each has its proper place and function.

Every living thing, including the cells in our bodies, strives to achieve a natural equilibrium, *homeostasis*. We tend, however, to be so preoccupied with the external world and meeting everyone else's expectations that we do little to restore the balance in our lives, until we are forced to by a life-threatening disease.

To restore this balance, we need to know who we are. We need to recognise that we are three people: the person we think we are, the person other people think we are, and the person we really are.

It's easy to recognise and think about the first two. We can define them and describe them. It is almost impossible to think about, let alone define, who we are unless we realise we are composed both of that of which we are aware and that of which we are unaware. We are, at one and the same time, something and nothing, being and non-being. As an ancient Chinese poem expresses it,

Many spokes unite to form the wheel –
but it is the centre that makes it useful.
We turn clay to make a vessel,
But it is where there is nothing that
the usefulness of it depends.
We cut doors and windows to make a house
But it is on those spaces where there is nothing that
the usefulness of the house depends.
Therefore just as we take advantage of what is,
we should recognise the usefulness of what is not.

To obtain balance, we need to honour both. We attend to our some-thingness when we take action, seek out the best medical attention, and strive to regain control over our lives. Our objective should also be to re-discover and experience the 'nothingness' or space in which we all reside. It will help you reach into your soul, draw strength from it, discover its healing power.

As the body and mind seem separate but are one, so something and nothing are part of one. We are so often deceived by what we see, and assume that if we see nothing, there is nothing. You can't see air, but you know it's there; you can't see thoughts, but whole civilisations have been built upon them. Metaphors make it easier to describe that which is beyond words or feelings. The unoccupied space in a room is what makes it habitable, so in music, the pauses between the notes give them meaning: if there were no pauses, there would be no music, merely noise. The tone and sound of a violin or a cello depends more on the hollow within the body than the wood from which it is made. A flute relies on its holes to produce its sounds. The stars and planets lean on the nothingness of space in order to reveal themselves. It is the space within us and within which we are – and over which we have no control – that is our true essence.

We can experience that state of nothingness and timelessness, our true soul, when we do nothing, and when we meditate in stillness, in that state of being that simply *is*. In the words of the mystic, Abraham Heschel, it is 'the secret stillness that precedes our birth and succeeds our death'.[8] Meditation and death are the doorways to nothingness. Meditation takes us back to that no-stress stage of our lives before we were born, when we were in nothingness, when there was balance and wholeness. Nothingness is the wise silence of the soul – that infinite, immeasurable, invisible, all-knowing stillness. We feel the awe of it, catch glimpses of its wonder, when we stand at the edges of the known. We often feel it in our hearts – that ineffable 'something' that is evoked when we listen to music, see a shaft of moonlight on the sea, listen to the words of a poem, gaze in awe at a distant star. The poet G.K. Chesterton captured the spirit of this when he wrote, 'There is a road from the eye to the heart that does not go through the intellect.' So did the poet and mystic, William Blake, when he wrote:

To see a World in a Grain of Sand
And a Heaven in a Wild Flower,
Hold Infinity in the palm of your hand
And Eternity in an hour.

We place interpretations on what our senses persuade us is the truth, but in the process lose sight of the fact that it is the soul that embraces and is in everything (what the philosopher Emerson calls the 'Over-Soul'), joins the known to the unknown, the somethingness to nothingness, and maintains a 'universe of unbroken wholeness'.[9]

Being and nothingness comprise a seamless all-ness, a one-ness. Some people refer to this as God – even though it is merely a word used to describe the indescribable; others call it that which cannot be named, the immeasurable, the Dreamtime, the collective unconscious.

Many scientists find it hard to acknowledge that the reason they have failed, will continue to fail, to confirm every unifying theory they present is because they cannot define God, the Over-Soul. With their emphasis on experimentation rather than revelation, it's not surprising that they steer clear of the word 'God'; for them it conjures up images of the irrational. For the scientist, the proof is in the contents of the pudding rather than in its taste, and so they are often unaware that the answers they seek do not lie outside us, are not observable through telescopes. They are obtained by looking inwards, through the revelation that comes from meditation. Those who have an aversion to the use of words such as 'intuition' or 'coincidence' fail to appreciate that there are different kinds of knowing.

Bringing it all together: prayer and meditation

What is prayer? Do we need it? If God is omniscient, omnipotent and omnipresent, then our thoughts, needs and expressed gratitude are already known; prayer is unnecessary. Perhaps we pray because we need to reach out, to bargain with a power greater than ourselves to deliver us from our suffering and the constant shock of reality.

We cannot speak and listen at the same time, so it is impossible to hear the voice of God when we pray, when we are focused on the words we are reading or uttering. It is only in meditation – prayer without words – that we can listen to the 'wee small voice' of the divine within us. As Psalm 46:9 says, 'Be still, and know that I am God.'

People talk of finding strength from 'somewhere'. In moments of crisis we pray, 'God, please grant me the strength to get through this ordeal.' Prayer is our acknowledgement that our strength to endure and our courage to forbear come from something or somewhere deep inside us – from a place we intuitively know is there. I believe that the indefinable 'something and somewhere' is the spirit of God that moves through everything, that teaches us the wisdom of patience and the reward of perfect courage which St Thomas Aquinas speaks of as a gift of the Divine Spirit. I also believe God speaks to us all the time – but that we don't hear – through nature, our bodymind, our instinct and our intuition.

A stone thrown into a pond makes a splash where it lands, and causes ripples that can be felt at some considerable distance. As you cannot discover the tranquillity that lies deep below the surface if you remain focused on the ripples, so you need to turn inwards to discover the peace within you to relieve the stresses that are affecting you.

We can re-discover this presence in the stillness of meditation, when we become aware of a 'merging' – a sense of 'expansiveness' in which we are a part of everything and, at the same time, everything is a part of us. In that moment, there is a deep awareness that your body and your mind are not separate – that you are, in a moment, both the seen and the seer, the knower and the known. As St Anthony said, 'The prayer of the monk is not perfect until he no longer realises himself, or the fact that he is praying.' It is how I would describe my own experience of meditation, and it is similar to what other people have told me they have experienced. We all agree it is an unsurpassable, ecstatic experience; we feel energised, humble, at peace, and wish for the afterglow to go on and on. Others have told me they can't meditate for fear of 'letting go' and losing control; that it feels as if they are dying.

When you meditate, your metabolic, heart and breathing rates slow down; sugar and lactate levels that rise when you are confronted by a 'fight-or-flight' situation are dramatically reduced. Moreover, brain waves also slow down, which explains why meditation is different from sleep, when brain waves remain active.

Can meditation cure cancer?

I do not believe that meditation can cure you of any disease. It can give your immune system time to listen to itself in an attempt to restore balance, but it cannot make rogue cells behave, nor is that its aim.

Meditation relaxes and soothes us, it teaches us to do one thing at a time, appreciate the moment in which we are, and that we have to experience nothingness for healing to occur. In this sense, the aim of healing is not to stay alive, but to become more whole, to find, as I believe Carl Jung correctly maintained, that the source of all true healing lies in bringing together the conscious and the unconscious – and that death is the ultimate healing.

That which occurred a second ago is history. That which will occur in a minute from now is conjecture. All we have is *now* – the point of the moment as it occurs. The best we can do is to respond to the moment – and the moment we do, we become aware of the oneness, comprised of being and nothing, that the mystic Joel Goldsmith aptly calls the 'Allness'.

How to meditate

If you have ever tried to meditate, you will know how hard it is to keep your thoughts from wandering, or to stop the itch that just won't go away. Instead of relaxing, you find yourself thinking about the very things you *don't* want to think about, find your thoughts uncontrollably running away from you.

You can train your mind, and as with physical exercise, it takes time before you see results. I urge you to start – and to persevere.

The meditations below are based on my own findings and those handed down over the centuries from all corners of the world. Remember, there is no one meditation that will suit everyone. If none of these methods suits you, look for one that does, but keep away from those people who ask for more than a nominal payment to teach you, especially those who would try to dissuade you from your faith, or tell you that their method is better than someone else's. You don't have to embrace a new faith or religion to practise meditation.

Studies have shown that noise over which we have no control is a stress factor that can lower our immune function.[10] Unless you have a soundproof room or can head for a cave, it's hard to find total quiet, so pick a time of day, perhaps early morning, when everything is at its quietest. In time, and with practice, you'll find you can meditate anywhere, no matter how noisy.

Pick a time and a place that suits you. Ask your wife, husband, partner or someone else to join you if you wish. Unplug the phone and switch on your voice mail. Set your alarm clock, or ask someone to tap you on the shoulder after a fixed time if you feel uncomfortable about drifting off for too long, or are worried you'll miss an appointment. With a little practice, you'll find you won't need to be alerted to come out of your meditation.

Start off with fifteen minutes a day, and extend it as you go. Don't set yourself any deadlines. For example, don't tell yourself you're going to increase it to half an hour by the end of the first week or to an hour by the end of second week, and so on.

There is no rule that says the more you meditate, the faster you'll heal, no law that says you have to do so at the same time every day, no edict that says you have to meditate alone. And there is no right way to sit, except that if you slouch you could end up with backache. You may find it easier to lie down if you are in pain or discomfort.

The objective is to achieve calmness, not agitation. When I was a child, my Zulu mentor taught me, 'Jwa. To be clever is be to be still.' I later interpreted this as an essential survival skill, as true for the hunter as for the hunted, for the healthy and those faced with cancer: if you want to live, stay still.

You may find these meditations difficult initially, and they can take time to master, but as you learn to stay focused you will find them easier.

Before you start

Sit comfortably on a chair or, if you choose or are confined to bed, place a single pillow under your head to keep your body as straight as possible. Some people find it helpful to place a small pillow or a rolled-up towel under each knee.

Stiffen your entire body as if your were clenching a fist, stay as rigid as you can, count slowly to five, then let go as you breathe out ever so slowly through your lips. While stiffening your body, notice how you tighten each of three sections of your body: chest and stomach; buttocks, thighs and calves; arms, shoulders, neck and eyes. Take two deep breaths, and clench your body again. Then repeat the procedure; three times in all. Let your breathing continue normally.

Use this technique before each meditation – or whenever you feel distressed and need to relax.

Meditations to focus

If you find it hard to be in the moment of the present without thinking about what happened yesterday or what you're going to do tomorrow, try the following three meditations to help you practise concentrating on one thing at a time.

CHEW A RAISIN

At the best of times, who notices what they eat? I mean, mouthful by mouthful?

'Chew your food a hundred times before you swallow,' my mother used to tell me. Her intention was good digestion, but her advice was equally good to help me focus on the moment. You really can't think of anything else as you count the munches.

Put a raisin in your mouth and count how many times you can chew it before there is nothing left. Taste its sweetness, its texture, its elasticity – and gently crunch the pips. Move it from one side of your mouth to the other, roll it round your tongue, press it against your palate and your front teeth. Play with it as if you never want to let it go.

If you don't like raisins, try a carrot or anything you like. The aim is not to eat, but to focus.

MEDITATIVE WALKING

Meditative walking is a centuries-old technique used by some Chinese monks to 'feel' the moment and achieve equilibrium. Find a smooth path, a part of your garden, a passageway at home and, preferably barefooted or with soft shoes, place the heel of one foot in front of the toes of the other, and start walking, the slower the better. Keep your arms in whatever position best helps you maintain balance. In time, you'll find you can do so with your palms pressed together in front of you resting against your chest. Feel the precise placement of your feet, the texture and inclination of the ground. Feel the ground under your feet. Feel how each step is one step more on a spiritual path, and that each step you take brings you closer to your true nature. How does it happen? It happens – all you have to do is take the first step.

LEAVES OF TIME

Close your eyes, and imagine yourself sitting or lying beside a gently flowing stream. Choose one you know, with pleasant associations, or dream up one that is ideal. Picture the stream meandering by from right to left.

It's autumn, the leaves have started to fall, and you can see them in all their glowing, autumnal colours – green, yellow, gold, brown.

One leaf drops onto the water and comes into view on the right. Look at it as it gently bobs and glides on the surface, at times floating smoothly, at other times whirling around in little eddies or as it gets trapped by a stone or reed, then breaks free and flows on.

Watch it carefully. Examine its texture, its colour, its shape. Watch it slowly flow away out of sight around a bend. Keeping your eyelids shut, turn your eyes again to the right, watch another leaf land, then gently glide into view. Examine it as it flows into your field of vision then, after about ten or twenty seconds, floats away out of sight.

Bear in mind, the more slowly the leaf glides by, the more you will break up the rapid and unending flow of thoughts that keep your mind so busy. If you notice your thoughts taking off in another direction, start again.

Meditation to relax

THE POND

Here is a relaxing meditation that will enable you to escape the agitation around you and to sink deep into yourself to re-experience the calmness and the nothingness of your soul.

Close your eyes. Picture yourself beside a pond or pool with ripples disturbing its surface. Step into the pond and keep wading in until the water closes over your head. Now imagine you are inside a large air bubble. Observe how the deeper you go, the calmer it gets.

Now you are so far removed from the disturbance above you, feel the water and your body merge as you adjust to the temperature of the water. As you keep sinking in your mini-sub bubble, the dappled light above you begins to fade until you cannot see anything around you. There is now nothing to disturb you. It is quiet and tranquil; the touch of the water against your skin is warm and reassuring. You notice a seat-shaped rock. Sit in it; stay for as long you wish. When you eventually choose to return to the surface and step out, notice how calm the surface of the pond has become – and how relaxed you feel.

BREATHING

Close your eyes. Start breathing normally. Notice how the air flows smoothly in and out of your nostrils. Feel the gentle rise and fall of your abdomen. Count each completed breath, and when you get to ten, start again. If you find your thoughts wandering or if you are distracted, start counting from one again. You may have to do this several times until you settle down.

Meditations for inner peace

EMPTINESS

Close your eyes. Picture the empty space in front of your face, between you and the wall. Every time you find your attention wandering off and you 'see' a place or a thing, imagine the space instead. Some people find it helpful to see the inside of their eyelids as a blank cinema screen, others imagine a point, a dot, in space midway between their eyes and focus on that.

STARSHIP

Close your eyes. Imagine yourself looking back at yourself. Feel yourself floating upwards, through the roof of your house and towards the sky. As you do, look down at yourself again, watch yourself growing smaller the further you drift away. You now have a bird's-eye view of your house, the street, the suburb and the town in which you live.

Keep drifting until you can see planet Earth getting smaller and smaller. Somewhere between earth and the moon, turn around and feel yourself heading out past the moon, each of the planets and the sun, until all you can see are stars.

As you fly through them, you notice they become fewer and fewer, until there are no more. You have arrived in empty space, and although you are still moving, there are no more reference points, so you feel as if you are still.

After a while (this can take about 20 minutes or more), the stars appear, one by one, until your universe is filled with them. In the distance you can see the distant sun and, as you get closer, the planets appear ahead of you.

Float past them until you see the earth, draw nearer and nearer until you can see the continents, the one in which you live, your city or town, your street, your house and, finally, you. Drift back into yourself and slowly open your eyes. Allow yourself a few minutes to adjust to your return. Take a deep breath. Open your eyes.

In this meditation, you may initially find it helpful to set your alarm clock to ring after about fifteen minutes as a signal to start your return journey home.

The way in which meditation puts us in touch with our spirit is beautifully described by Kahlil Gibran in *The Prophet*,

You are not encased within your bodies,
nor confined to the houses or fields.
That which is you dwells above the mountain...
a thing free, a spirit that envelopes the earth
and moves in the ether.

thirteen

living in the
face of death

'The most beautiful experience
we can have is the mysterious.'

ALBERT EINSTEIN

A life-threatening disease such as cancer stops you in your tracks, compels you, as nothing else does, to find an explanation for the predicament in which you now find yourself. You may want life to be what it was like before your diagnosis but, every day in hundreds of little ways, you discover that it can never be the same, that nothing can bring back yesterday or what happened one minute ago. Cancer says that life can never be as it was, or as you want it to be. *Life can only be as it is.*

Most people granted a reprieve eventually come to see that their disease has given them a second chance to re-experience life. Almost all of the people I know – including me – who have ever recovered from cancer feel that their lives have changed for the better, that they now have their priorities right and, for the first time, have the balance that was lacking. They also find death more acceptable, dying less frightening, and are thankful they have been granted the chance to complete their unfinished business.

Cancer can be less frightening if, instead of seeing it as a Grim Reaper, you view it as a messenger of Fate shaking you out of your complacency, challenging you to face your fears, daring you to do the things you've always wanted to do, asking you to serve others selflessly, or in any number of ways persuading you that life is worth the struggle. Meet the challenge, and your quality of your life will improve. You may even live longer.

You will reduce your chances of learning all this from your experience if you carry on with your life much as you did before, and regard healing and cure in the same light. Quality of life, cure and healing are all linked, but they are not the same. It's one thing to have fewer symptoms or to be symptom-free – it's quite another to have peace of mind; one thing to be told you no longer require treatment – quite another to feel as if your life is unfulfilled. Medicine may restore your health, but only you can achieve the healing of your spirit that comes when you feel at ease with yourself and the world around you, are free to love and be loved, and can say, 'I feel alive.'

Most people want to try to make sense of what life is all about, and what their role is in the scheme of things, but all too often are consumed by the ordinary and the everyday. 'I don't have time to think about such matters,' they say. A life-threatening disease compels you to look at life from a completely different point of view. Ordinary events become extra-ordinary, you now appreciate the things you took for granted, find previous priorities no longer hold you in their grip.

I do not wish to romanticise disease or the prospect of death, but I believe it takes a cataclysmic event to rouse most of us out of our indifference to life. Cancer is an earthquake; it shifts us from a state of complacency to one of wonderment, from blindly following rituals to actively pursuing the spiritual, from being a passive spectator of life to being an active participant in it. Woody Allen once said, 'I know I have to die, but I don't want to be there when it happens.' We all know that nature must win in the end: cancer compels us to accept this. It also gives us some time in which to do so.

Understand the past to prepare for the future

As your doctor takes note of your medical history in order to work out how to treat you, so you need to examine your past to help you live in the present, without fear of the future. It's like learning to walk again; you have to learn new skills.

When we were children we wanted to be loved by our parents, and remain the focus of their constant attention. We learned at a very early age that it was more rewarding, safer and far less painful to do what we were told, even if it meant doing the opposite of what we really wanted to do. We also learned that the benefit of not answering back and doing as we were told was to be called a good child. These tactics saved us from every child's worst fears: emotional and physical abandonment.

We accepted, without question, that everything done to and for us was for our own good. And so the pattern was set for us to go through life acting out a part, a role, according to a script written by our parents, our teachers, society at large. Afraid of the consequences of revealing ourselves, we keep the wise child within us hidden from view, and in the process take on an inauthentic role and remain out of balance, out of sync, no longer whole. The result is that we are split into three: the person we have become by adjustment, the person others think we are, and the one we really are and have now forgotten. It may be that our yearning to find the divine source of everything is an attempt to connect with who we once were – a wise child, full of understanding and intuition buried under a mountain of expectation.

Our bodymind is aware of the tear in its fabric, between who we are and want to be and who other people want us to be. And so the conflict begins. The seeds of disquiet and dis-ease are sown. Think back to anything that has happened in your life, and you will recall the accompanying feeling of unease you felt when you were asked to do something that 'didn't feel right', 'went against the grain', or 'rubbed you up the wrong way' – and how you never spoke up, never said, 'No.'

If you can imagine that you have spent your whole life doing what didn't feel right, holding in your feelings and making compromises, you will realise how right the words are of Albert Schweitzer, doctor and Nobel Prize winner, when he said, 'The tragedy of life is what dies inside a man while he lives.'

The differences in the ways we were raised as children reveal themselves in so many ways. Those who were 'dumping grounds' for their parents' failures rarely have a positive view of their own lives. Those whose dreams were nurtured – no matter how far-fetched they appeared to their parents' vision – rarely flinch from life's challenges. Those who were constantly reminded by their parents of plans scuttled and 'sacrifices' made on their behalf often feel guilty, and hardly ever succeed in life: to achieve success would be to accentuate their parents' *lack* of success. Those who have been told by their parents from an early age to 'grow up' and 'stop acting like a child' lose their childish spontaneity, find life a grind and, in deference to their parents' caveats, find little joy in anything they do.

There is a myth that maturity means surrendering your youthful fantasies and ceasing to dream. I believe we bury the very life-force our dreams engender from the moment we stop asking and seeking, put occupational success and responsibility ahead of personal growth, find it easier to 'take it easy' rather than to demand more of ourselves.

I speak from the heart on these matters. They are what I had to contend with, and are common threads running through all the dialogues with people I have counselled. You can start the healing process of your bodymind by recovering your dream and listening to the 'wee small voice' of your wise, inner child – the voice of the divine. The process may take years, and it often does, but if you are committed to its pursuit, you could survive long enough to realise it.

A life with purpose is one in which you respect each level of your being – from the child at your core to the nervous 'about-to-be-reborn' person you now are. Life is much more interesting when you seek to fulfil your dreams because they reflect what *you* want – not what others expect of you. Life is rarely humdrum – more likely to be extra-ordinary – when you follow the irrational calling of your spirit from within, or in the words of Carl Jung, 'Anyone with a vocation hears the voice of the inner man.'[1] Perhaps the easiest way to understand yourself is simply to be yourself.

Healing the rift

Cancer changes everything, and everyone. It allows us to cut out the dead wood in our life – people, relationships, unnecessary obligations – and focus on what we want, perhaps for the first, and maybe the last, time in our life. Cancer puts an end to the inauthentic lives we lead when, instead of meeting other people's expectations and fulfilling our obligations to them, we now respond to our own.

'Cancer made me feel legitimate,' said Margaret, a woman I counselled. No one else I know has described this so aptly.

What this means is that a life-threatening disease *gives you permission to be who you are*. What people expect of you as a cancer patient is not only quite different from what they expect from other people, but from who you were before you were diagnosed. So, if you can get past the point where you are attempting to make a recovery for the sake of other people – including your parents, your spouse, your children or your grandchildren – you can become legitimate, authentic.

You take a gigantic leap towards achieving your own healing when you say, 'I'm sick of being sick!' It is only when you are driven to exasperation by your cancer rather than your fear of it, when you realise that your disease is no longer serving your best interests, and when you know there is nothing more anyone else can do for you – in short, when you have reached what seems to be rock bottom – that you realise the truth of the old Chinese saying: 'By being pained at the thought of having the disease, we are preserved from it.'

You can achieve a breakthrough in healing when you eventually choose to stop 'doing' something about your disease as if it were something outside of yourself and choose to 'be' who you are. You can't do this if you are trying to meet the needs of others; when you still say, for example, 'After all they've done for me, I owe it to everyone around me to recover,' or 'I suppose I should try and get better; my children need me.' It has been my experience that those who make these comments seldom recover. If, on the other hand, you choose to live the rest of your life according to who you really are, you will be acting legitimately and with purpose. It is the most important life-promoting gift you can receive from a cancer diagnosis.

Meditation to reclaim your self

Close your eyes. Get comfortable on a chair or bed, relax yourself as I described in the previous chapter.

In your mind's eye, imagine you're looking through your photograph album and come across your favourite picture of yourself at any age up to eight. Now, imagine you are the photographer taking that picture, are present at the moment it was taken.

Put your camera down, walk over to yourself as a child, pick him or her up, and cradle him or her in your arms. Say, ' I have come back for you. I never really went away. I'm sorry, but I forgot all about you. I missed you – but now I will never let you go.' Hold that child close to you. Feel the texture of his or her skin against your face, and kiss his or her cheek. Say, 'You'll be safe now. I'll take care of you forever. I won't forget you again, ever.'

Hold that child for as long as you can, then put him or her down, and say, 'I'll come back for you. Don't worry. Everything is OK now.'

Walk back to your camera, pick it up, look through the viewfinder, see the same photograph in your album. Close the album. Open your eyes.

Any time you feel unsure about making any decision, are 'out of sync' or distressed, repeat this meditation. It's the most healing one I know.

How time governs our lives

We are so mesmerised by time that when we are told we have a life-threatening disease, our first question is usually, 'How much time have I got left?'

In that one urgent question, you reveal that, perhaps even more than your fear of death, you fear 'losing time'. Suddenly, you feel trapped in the cage of time, believe that when there is no more time, there will be no more of you. When a doctor tells you that you have six months to live, the hex he puts on you is one of time, not death. Yet death and time are so linked, people who believe they are dying say, 'My time's up,' as the convict is not sentenced to jail, but to 'six months'.

We have come to view time as a resource, something to be managed and measured as if we can impose our will on it. If we don't manage time well, we say we don't have enough of it to spare to visit family and friends, to go on holidays. We turn down invitations by saying, 'I don't have the time.' We are irritated by people who 'waste time' or seem to have 'time on their hands'. The ultimate regard we have for time as a resource is reflected in the statement, 'Time is money.' The irony is that no matter how many times you wind your watch or replace its battery, you have no control over time. This is so obvious, yet we 'watch' time on our wrists, on the clocks beside our beds, and continually ask, 'How much time do I have?', 'Am I on time?' or exclaim 'I haven't got any time,' 'I'm running out of time.'

We are so obsessed with time, the more we feel the loss of it, the more anxious, desperate and hopeless we get. I understand this well.

Before my first cancer diagnosis, I was killing myself trying to find time for this and that. No matter how well I planned things, there was never enough time. When I realised I had really run out of time, the things I had once valued I now found trivial – and vice versa.

In our pursuit of material wealth, raising our children and acquiring possessions, we never seem to have enough time for ourselves. We become oblivious to the wonders of nature, lose sight of the value and importance of relationships, 'waste' time by being spectators rather than participants in life.

A life-threatening disease throws up a seemingly endless list of things to do. In a panic, you realise that what once seemed so easy to defer is now urgent. Indeed, there may be little time left to tidy up your personal and business affairs; people with whom you needed to repair broken links and heal wounded feelings may have died or moved away. You could be left with the feeling there are still things that need to be done, but now cannot be done. You may feel that your disease has overtaken you and, in the process, denied you the opportunity to fulfil your potential. There are many people who look back on their lives and say, 'If only I had done this or that, stayed here, gone there…' The epitaph on the grave of a hypochondriac reads, 'I told you so.' The memorial to an unlived life reads, ' If only…'

You may express your fear about what appears to you as an all-too-short future by saying, 'If only I could live to see my children growing up,' or 'If only I had time to do that.' I believe we fear time because of our fear of losing the life we never led, or that there is no time left to fulfil our potential, realise our long-lost dreams. The fear of a wasted life presents an awesome prospect.

There is no better time than now to complete all your 'if-only's – saying your farewells, drawing up a will, signing a living will, patching up old differences and grievances. You cannot be free to make the most of whatever life you have left as long as these issues are unresolved. If you still feel there are things to be done, there are. If you think you've done everything, you haven't. If you think there's nothing more you can do, there is.

As with other life-threatening diseases, cancer is a messenger who has come to remind us that this life is part of a spiritual journey, that our mission is not to acquire wealth but wisdom, and to help others.

Those who realise that this is a spiritual journey strive to give added meaning to their lives, find expression in various creative acts, give top priority to completing their unfinished business.

Living in the present

It seems to me that our view of time affects the way we handle a crisis which, in turn, can determine our survive-ability.

Professor Schwartz, of the University of Massachusetts Medical School, has found that we have an inbuilt time-keeping mechanism, the suprachiasmatic nucleus behind the optic nerve, that ensures our body rhythms stay in phase with the earth's rotation and alternation of day and night. When we are out of phase, we say we are 'out of sync'. The symptoms are real: insomnia, jet lag, fatigue, moodiness, stomach upset.

Our bodies are so exquisitely sensitive to this rhythm that our immune system also responds accordingly. Doctors know this well. For example, the efficacy and side effects of drugs are greatly affected by the time of day they are administered. A drug supposed to be taken in the morning will not be as effective if taken at night; stress hormone levels will vary at different times of the day; asthma sufferers require a long-acting drug to cope with their varying breathing patterns; most cases of cardiac arrest occur in late morning.[2]

Our perception of time is even more variable, and linked with our emotional life. For example, when we are engaged in a task we are unwilling to do, or find boring, time seems to drag; when we enjoy what we're doing, are preoccupied, time seems to fly.

In fact, it is only our varying perceptions of time that differ; real time doesn't change. Time *is*. Time does not 'happen'. It is always present. It makes no sense to say that the less we do, the more time we have; or the more we do, the less time we have. All we can really say is that it *seems* as if we have more or less time, as the case may be.

We need to live in the present moment to heal and achieve wholeness. This does not mean sitting passively in a chair and doing nothing, even meditating all day. It means living as you did when you were a three-year-old child, enjoying every moment, unconcerned with what will happen next, or what happened earlier. Living in the moment does not imply hedonism or acquiring possessions since they are fleeting, but rather looking into the nature of things, seeing time in the here and now, and finding freedom from the restraint of past regrets and future fears. If we can stop seeing time as a thing or a resource, then the future is no longer a set of unfulfilled time, the past not simply a pile of used-up time.

Accept the present as an ongoing moment, and you will realise it is irrelevant to wonder about the treatment you've had, what its likely effects will be, whether your disease will recur, or whether you will get another cancer. Constantly thinking of what will happen to you next is to live in an imaginary future instead of living in the here and the now – in wholeness, being together, mind and body, here and now, present to yourself and to others. At best, as human beings, we can use our brain's larger cortex to change our perceptions so we can understand more of what is happening.

To gain perspective on this view, you need to see yourself as the object of your intellectual curiosity: it's the key to survival. It's finding the balance that comes when you step back, see yourself as something separate, and make a choice without prejudice. You can do it if you're free of unresolved internal conflicts, and not driven by unconscious fears. The secret is knowing when to hold on or let go, allowing intuition and reason to honour each other's right to make decisions on your behalf, and without censure from each other. You know intuition and instinct are at work when, at times, the harder you try to maintain control, the more you lose it; and sometimes the more laid-back you are, the more things fall your way. Balance and wholeness come when you realise, finally, that you can't hold onto life indefinitely, and that you can't lose it when you die.

In order to achieve wholeness, all we have to do is let go of our vain belief that we can alter natural laws. The moment we surrender this, we are freed to concentrate on the moment that is now, and as Emerson said, 'To fill the hour – that is happiness.'

Instead of being trapped in the cage of time, we have to see the past and the future as part of the vast open field of the present, for only then can we see we are always on the way to becoming something else, that everything is in transition and that, as Wordsworth said,

Though nothing can bring back the hour
Of splendour in the grass, of glory in the flower,

We will grieve not, rather find
Strength in what remains behind.

Aim for a goal

Some people question the notion that we should attempt to alter our destiny, believe that as we are programmed by biological factors we should accept whatever fate throws at us and bow to the inevitable. I don't agree with this view. I believe that if we respond to life, anything becomes possible. We have to act as if destiny does not affect our freedom of choice.

As *natural* beings we are restrained by natural laws; as *human* beings we have freedom to exercise our will. Caught between spiritual freedom and outward destiny, we must again and again decide which direction to take. Taking or avoiding a particular course of action requires weighing up the risks and taking responsibility for the choice you make. Making choices is a continual process; it's the way in which we give meaning to the struggle and uniqueness of life. Only by making choices can we maximise our freedom. It means we have to seriously question the integrity of doctors who choose to tell us how long we have to live and ask: does their statement reflect *our* destiny or *theirs*?

Accepting responsibility for freedom of choice can turn a life-threatening disease into a starting-point rather than an end-point of the challenge facing you. I believe that every moment of our lives represents a new beginning, all of life a demand that we respond to it.

How to set goals

Keep in mind that the goals you set yourself are not the end, rather intermediate points on the path to your ultimate recovery. They should be manageable goals, enabling you to deal with life in bite-size pieces that can be chewed on and savoured. This will create a sense of action and purpose, of being able to achieve something, rather than being left with a sense of helplessness. Of course, you have to picture an outcome, just as in any ball game, you have to decide where you want the ball to go – then focus on it and nothing else, or else you'll miss.

Take a sheet of paper, draw two columns on it. Head one column, 'Can do now', head the other column, 'Can't do now'.

Under the heading 'Can't do now' list those things you *can't* imagine achieving in the immediate future because you're still undergoing treatment, recovering from it, and are still too weak. For example, you may list such things as: lay down a new kitchen floor – paint the house – visit friend overseas – give up job and do what I really want to do – start a new hobby.

Under the heading 'Can do now' list those things you *can* imagine doing in the immediate future, and then set about doing them, one by one. For example, under this heading you may list such issues as: finish reading this book – start a journal – read up more about my disease – walk for twenty minutes each day – make an appointment with my lawyer and accountant to discuss my affairs – bury the hatchet with old Bob down the road – have dinner at my favourite restaurant – learn to meditate – try to be more tolerant and a better listener (to my husband, wife, parent, son or daughter, as the case may be). You may find that putting them in order of importance will enable you to deal with the more difficult issues first, so the rest becomes a breeze.

When you've worked your way through the 'Can do now' list, start on the 'Can't do now' one, but change the title of it to 'Can do now', and start a new 'Can't do now' list.

Most people try to do everything at once, and usually fail. Again, the issue is one of time, trying to crowd everything into one moment. Draw up these lists, and you'll become task-oriented rather than time-oriented. And you'll find the courage to change the things you can.

The fact that you have cancer doesn't mean the world out there is going to change for you, or that people are necessarily going to treat you differently from the way they did before. However, when you change, you will immediately create a sense of your own possibilities – and the mere fact of doing something will make you feel good about yourself. So focused, you'll find yourself free to live in the continuing present. 'Take care of today and tomorrow will take care of itself' was never a more appropriate proverb than now.

Here's something else to consider: the only way to imagine an end to this period in your life is to change your view of it, and you will the moment you say 'when' instead of 'if'.

Say to yourself, '*When* I have done this I will do that,' rather than, 'I will do that *if* I get through this.'

Say, '*When* my treatment has stopped I will draw up a "Can do" and "Can't do" list.' Don't say, '*If* I get through the treatment I will draw up the lists.'

Substitute 'when' for 'if', and you will help to change your attitude from passive to active; no longer will you see yourself as someone having things done to you. The word 'when' creates a sequence; the word 'if' puts everything on hold.

To move past your illness, you have to start somewhere. Robert Schuller, internationally known American churchman, reminds us of this when he says, 'Winning starts with beginning, and beginning starts with a single action.'[3] The decision you make today will be a reality tomorrow; as a painting starts with a single brush stroke, start redrawing your life. You may not be able to picture all of your future right now, but with each stroke it will become clearer and clearer, as long as you don't give up.

How to break the spell of time

By living in the continuing present you can break the spell of your doctor's prediction that you are going to die at a clock-determined time. When I was told I had leukemia, I became 'frozen in time'. With no prospect of a future, the best I could do was to manage the moment – and the moment I did I became focused on the next moment and the next. I have no doubt that living in the moment helped to dispel my fear of time, and of death.

Richard Byrd, the famous Arctic explorer, who was isolated in his polar camp, experimented with new ways to live in the present. His goal was to achieve 'full mastery of the impinging moment'. To do so, he shut out the past and concentrated on those activities that would have meaning for the moment. He set himself achievable and visible goals: to cook more quickly, to take more accurate weather observations, to do things more systematically.[4]

Here are some things you can do:

- To gain more time, start doing those things that take more time.
- To stop reminding yourself that time is fleeting, lock your watch away. If you're worried about missing your next doctor's

appointment, ask her to call you the day before your
appointment to remind you.

☞ Enhance your appreciation of the present – which is all we
have – by doing those things that keep you in the present,
whatever they are: meditation, gardening, knitting,
needlepoint, and keeping a journal.

☞ Certainly, there is no better time than now to start doing those
things you've always wanted to do. It's what survivors do. If
your reply to this is a concerned, 'But will I have enough time
to finish what I start?' my answer is, 'Yes, you will – *if* you
forget the old way of thinking about time and re-invent a new
time-*less* framework for yourself.' Don't count the days; make
the days count.

In such a model, no matter what task you set for yourself, all you can
do – and all you need to do – is to start now. In any journey, the most
important step you take is the first, since the completion of any task
lies beyond this moment and is, therefore, out of your control.

Mountain climbers, for example, focus on each step at each
moment. They know that a moment's distraction can be fatal.

My story

Much of what I have spoken about is reflected in my own story.

Until my diagnosis, everything I had ever done had been focused
on what I was going to do next. 'You're only as good as your next project' was the underlying message I had lived with for almost 20 years
in the world of advertising. But now my future was gone. I was
stranded in the realisation that all I had was now, and that no one else
could face this moment for me.

I was released from the grip of that frozen moment as soon as I
remembered the wisdom handed to me by our Zulu housekeeper,
John Ndmande, when I was a child. From the distant past I heard his
voice telling me,

*Jwa, impi [Zulu warrior] must be clever if he wants to live. When he
is out hunting, armed only with his assegai [short, stabbing spear] and
shield, he always watches out for his back. You must make sure the
wind is blowing towards you. The simba [lion] must never smell you.*

Intuitively I knew that I had to rely on myself to gain an advantage. In the process of tracking down my foe, I was compelled to hone my hunting skills, to discover what I could and couldn't do, and to face my deepest fears. If there was any uncertainty left in me, it was my recollection of the second of John Ndmande's lessons that provided me with the emotional and spiritual strength to cope with what lay ahead. 'To be clever is to be still.'

Instinctively I realised that there was little else I could do but manage the moment. As soon as I did, I became focused on the next moment, and the next, and the next. I had discovered the continuing present of being in the mindful moment. Never one to leave anything to chance, I also went for a second opinion.

Later, as I struggled through the side effects of treatment, I recalled another old Zulu saying John had taught me, 'Unless you go through hard times you cannot be a man.'

Denial of death

In the Western world, the promise of science enables most people to live in denial of death (see Chapter 10). Some draw comfort from the fact that some body parts can be replaced, and that vitamins, micronutrients and anti-oxidants may eventually halt the ageing, dying process. Others see their lives as on a movie screen, where everything is youth-oriented and expendable.

I believe we ought always to strive to maximise our potential, but with everyone so centred on being better and more successful, we have allowed little room for making mistakes, even less for failure. Not surprisingly, when we fail – and it is a part of the human condition that we will, often – we do not know how to cope. Those around us have also never been taught how to deal with failure, so they are of little or no help in comforting us when we slip or falter; we and they feel let down. And when we are handed a life-threatening diagnosis, and face the prospect of failing to beat death, we are mortified.

Life and death are, have always been, a heartbeat apart, yet people react with such shock and horror to being told they have a life-threatening disease, it is apparent they are unprepared for it. Their response may even turn to unbridled fear if their belief system hints at consequences after life too dire to contemplate.

Some say, 'I'll worry about it when the time comes.' Others say, 'I don't want to think about it.' Most people say, 'If I'm going to die, I want it to be quick. And I don't want to know about it.'

To wish for a sudden death for which you have had no time to prepare is like emigrating to a new country without knowing anything – about its climate, politics or history. As the moment of death finally approaches, most people find themselves regretting that they had not given more thought to the purpose of life, that they have not come to terms with their death, and now feel 'rushed' and angry.

I believe that the end of this life is at one and the same time our embarkation and re-entry point for our onward journey. As such, we ought to be devoting more of our time and energies towards preparing for the take-off. In Buddhism, monks are taught the words of the Buddha, 'Death comes unexpectedly. How can we bargain with it?' We have no idea when our flight will be called, we can't choose our seat or take any baggage. And we have to fly alone. With our God-given gifts of intellect, imagination and wisdom, and living in a conscious world that demands we attempt to find the reason for our existence, we have been granted a unique opportunity to arrive at the moment of transition at least as wise as when we arrived, at our birth.

One of the major criticisms levelled at most religions is that they are too focused on the after-life, neglectful of this one. Certainly, there has to be a balance. To fail to witness the wonders of this life is to fail to appreciate that as death imbues life with meaning, so life imbues death with meaning. It seems so many people go through life without being aware of this balance, and that the spirit that moves through everything demands we live life for it, not die for it.

We cannot imagine what life would be like if it had no end, yet it is only by persuading ourselves of the value of life that we can effectively keep our fear of death under control. We can only fear death if we have not lived life in the moment, emptied the contents of our baggage, said our farewells, and not embraced the love of the divine spirit within us, and within which we are.

Why we have to die in order to live

It is our awareness that our existence at this level is finite that compels us to give meaning to life. It is why we have created the civilisations we have. If we believe we will live forever, there will be no need to be remembered, or to prepare for an uncertain future, so there will no be need for art, poetry, music, trade, industry or commerce. In the light of a never-ending existence, no problem, challenge or change would ever be considered important enough to require our attention; we would procrastinate *ad infinitum*. In this sense, death is life's solution to laziness.

We also know that where there is no change, there is boredom. Life as we know it is finite – much as we may fear it and prefer not to think about it – but that is what gives it its unique quality. It is brevity of life that presses us into service, makes us want to savour every moment to the fullest of our abilities. Without death, life would be meaningless. As Bruno Bettelheim reflected, 'The only antidote to death is to find meaning in life, yet it is death which gives life its deepest and most unique meaning.'[5]

What's the point of suffering?

It may be hard for you right now to accept that you cannot truly understand or appreciate what life is all about unless you have suffered.

Most people tend to see suffering in the abstract; it's what other people undergo and, for much of the time, it is associated with deprivation, such as lack of food, love, the loss of someone close. Sufferers exclaim, 'Why do I have to suffer like this?';'Why me?'. They ask these questions as if suffering were always unfair and, if it cannot be prevented, should be eliminated as quickly as possible. Modern medicine has helped to relieve suffering associated with physical pain, but mental anguish and spiritual suffering remain a hurdle for those who seek peace of mind and improved quality of life.

I suggest that just as we have good days and bad days, and we can't really appreciate one without the other, so we cannot appreciate the magical and blissful moments of life without experiencing suffering.

'But why should innocent people have to suffer?' you ask. Are you not an innocent? Do you deserve to suffer?

I believe that life demands we gain as much knowledge and wisdom as we can in preparation for the next part of our journey. The suffering of others teaches us compassion, opens our hearts to a greater understanding, and makes us less fearful of suffering. As Kahlil Gibran, the mystic and poet, wrote, 'The deeper that sorrow carves into your being, the more joy you can contain. Is not the cup that holds the wine the very cup that was burned in the potter's oven? And is not the lute that soothes your spirit the very wood that was hollowed with knives?'

If you regard suffering as unnatural, you will regard life itself as unnatural, and therefore one big mistake; if you believe suffering is for nothing, life is meaningless. But if our suffering can raise our awareness of our spirituality, we can, I believe, come to view cancer as the messenger who has called our attention to the fact that all is not well, that we have reached a crossroad, that we have to take a new direction to complete this leg of our spiritual journey.

All too often we are intimidated by cancer's physical presence, and see it as an awesome foe to whom we must bow our heads in surrender, without realising the challenge we face is to overcome the tentacled monster and retrieve the treasure of life. It is the reward of the hero's journey when, after setting out and enduring much hardship along the way, he finally slays the dragon, retrieves the treasure and returns it to his people.

Some people would appear better able to face the hero's journey than others; many are overwhelmed by their fears, and stay rooted to the spot. However, there are many, and I hope you are one of them, who are awakened by the growl of the monster, and rise to the challenge knowing that even heroes die. You cannot ignore suffering; you have to go through it. The greatest courage you can show is the courage to suffer, and endure.

Life after death

I closed my eyes, relaxed my body, and began to meditate when suddenly, I felt myself falling. This seemed strange as I was not falling downwards, but forwards, and then, before I knew it, found myself floating down a long, dark tunnel with a faint light in the distance.

I drifted towards it in slow motion not making contact with the sides. I had no bodily sensations at all. At first I was frightened, but as I drew nearer, my trepidation began to ease and I was curious about what lay ahead. The brightness grew so intense it almost blinded me, and as I finally emerged from the tunnel into what I can only describe as total whiteness, I was surrounded by it. I was in it; it was in me; and I was a part of it. The light became even more brilliant so I could see nothing except the whiteness. It had a clarity that was startling. There was neither up nor down, no left, no right. I floated, wrapped in a cloud of whiteness. I was flooded with an incredible sense of love and peace. I felt boundless and without edges. No voice spoke, yet I knew this was death, that I was alive in a different kind of way, and it was OK. There was nothing to fear. I didn't want to leave, but although nothing was said, I knew I had to return and tell what had happened. Suddenly I felt myself hurtling back along the tunnel, the light receding to a vanishing point. I have no idea how long I remained in what seemed to be an eternity of light. Then my eyes opened. Ahead of me, through a window, I could see a blue sky. I had returned.

I was at a loss to explain it, yet in that moment I knew I had experienced something quite extraordinary and beautiful. I felt overwhelmed with joy. For the first time since I was a child, my fear of dying had gone. Instead, I felt a sense of awe, acceptance and serenity. I wondered if I had been hallucinating, but I was on no drugs, had simply been meditating, letting go of everything. A few months later, I had a second, similar encounter. On this occasion, I experienced a slightly different feeling. It was wordless and yet it had a voice, and I knew that this was what it was going to be like when I died – and that this is what it's like to be with God.

Had I hallucinated twice? Had my imagination compensated for my dread of dying, or was this an adjustment to prepare me for death? A week later, I attended an Elisabeth Kübler-Ross seminar, and I felt myself go cold as she described how, in her research, similar experiences had been related to her by people who had been through what she called 'a near-death experience'. I was reassured I wasn't going mad, when she added that she believed near-death experiences proved there was life after death.

The literature on near-death experiences (NDEs)[6] is studded with expressions used by various authors to explain away this phenomenon: increased brain activity, oxygen deprivation, raised endorphin levels, a desire to find a utopian society, social and personal betterment, secular salvation. Some authors have suggested that NDEs are located in that part of the brain that is associated with our unconscious desires and ability to dream; others say they reflect an affective disorder known as 'depersonalisation' used by people to cushion death's blow to the ego or help you plan a course of action to survive; still others refer to NDEs as altered states of consciousness, and ask whether consciousness transcends physical or bodily death.

I don't see my NDE as fitting any of the above descriptions, yet if it *is* a dream, is it any less real? I could just as easily have had a nightmare, but I didn't. Our dreams, no less than meditation, are our doorway to eternity, to the collective unconscious, to God. If anything, I see NDEs as an added confirmation that there is a divine being, that we exist as part of it, are aware of it consciously and unconsciously, and that birth and death, as with many other events, are our rites of passage through life eternal. Through my experience, I came to see that God is all light, and that we are so dazzled and blinded by its brilliance, that nothing specific can be seen. It is only here, in this reality, where the light is less intense and there are shadows to help us differentiate what we can see, that we can gaze in awe at God's creations.

People who return from their vacations and adventures are usually excited about their experiences, and want to share them with everyone. Rarely does anyone question the truth of what they say, and often base the choice of their next journey on what they have heard. I feel the same way about my two NDEs. I am aware that some religions regard this subject as taboo, but just as I find it just as hard to avoid the subject of death when talking about cancer, so I find it is impossible to avoid the subject of life after death.

A wonderful tale illustrates the concept that our exit from the womb is the birth of the body, and the exit from the body the re-birth of the soul to eternal life.

A set of twins starts growing in the safety and warmth of their mother's womb. Their watery world is all they know, but as time passes they begin to wonder what will happen when they depart their blissful surroundings.

The first child believes that a new life awaits him as a being with uncramped arms and legs, able to eat thorough his mouth, hear through his ears and see vast distances with his eyes. The second child dismisses his brother's ideas by telling him that all he is doing is calming his fear of death through fanciful use of his imagination. With all the confidence of the ignorant, he states, 'There will be an end to consciousness. There will be nothing, just a black void.'

Suddenly there is a loud, tearing sound, and the believing brother disappears.

The second child is so shocked by the sudden turn of events, he falls silent. In the distance he hears a scream followed by a loud roar.

'It's worse than I thought,' he mutters to himself. 'The end is terrible.' However, the sceptical brother soon discovers that the shriek was a sign of his brother's first breath, and the shouting the chorus of congratulations from the doctors and nurses and the parents looking on.[7]

You never know

When you've gone round after round with pain, discomfort and incapacity; when you've been rocked back on your heels by a barrage of chemotherapy, radiotherapy or other treatments, you can be excused for asking, 'Why go on?'

Only you can answer that question, but before you decide to throw in the towel, I would ask you to weigh up the possibilities that may still lie ahead if you consider, as psychiatrist and author Viktor Frankl did when he was imprisoned in a concentration camp during World War II, that 'no man can ever know what life still holds in store for him, or what magnificent hour may still await him.'[8]

My late father was fond of relating a Russian tale from the turn of the century about a farmer's son who went out riding one day and returned with a herd of wild horses he had found. Their neighbour heard the news and came to congratulate the farmer on his windfall.

'What incredible luck!' he exclaimed.

'Well, you never know,' replied the farmer.

A few days later, while trying to break them in, the son was thrown by one of the horses and broke his leg. Their neighbour heard what had happened and came to offer his sympathy.

'What bad luck,' he said.

'Well, you never know,' replied the farmer.

Conscription was in force at the time, and sure enough, a week after the accident, an army officer arrived with call-up papers for the son to serve on the Eastern front where there was every chance he would be killed. When he saw the broken leg, he revoked the orders. Their neighbour heard the good news and came to wish them well.

'You son is so lucky!'

'Well, you never know,' replied the farmer.

You also never know what fate has in store for you. Your worst fears may never be realised. Keep this story in mind and you may find it easier to cope. You may feel hopeful one day, full of gloom the next; you never know.

'Why go on?' Well, you aren't dead until you're dead, so as long as you can breathe, you can never tell what will happen next.

Celebrate the struggle

The philosopher Wittgenstein maintained that 'that whereof one cannot speak, thereof must one be silent.' In the face of a life-threatening disease, I find it hard *not* to talk about God.

In my view, there is no person or 'someone out there' you can call God. To describe God in a rational way implies that the same reference points that apply to us also apply to that which cannot be named. The way to approach God is not through reason, but through a leap of faith that transcends the logical and the empirical. We can intellectualise anything we like about the meaning of life and death and how life began and why, but we can never grasp their significance until we open the door to intuition and faith. The fact that we experience them in one way or another gives their intangibility substance.

I believe that God is everywhere, and in everything. Just as I am in God, so God is in me. The knower and the known are synchronous; the observer and the observed are co-existent. The universe is a harmonious whole and it's here, staring us in the face like the man who mislaid his spectacles, looks here, there and everywhere, then discovers he was wearing them all the time. Eternity is in the moment.

Science has come close to making sense of this through quantum theory, although some scientists still argue about the details. It was Einstein's work into the nature of light that led Niels Bohr, Louis DeBrogli, Werner Heisinger, Erwin Schrödinger, Wolfgang Pauli and Paul Dirac to formulate an atomic theory that holds that particles can travel like waves, and waves like particles. What this means is that particles can jump from point to point, occupy several places at once, and 'communicate' at the speed of light. This is possible only if one sees empty space and matter as one.

In 1964, a physicist, John Bell, proposed a theorem confirming Einstein's original theory and now known as Bell's Theorem. It indicates that when two particles, once in contact with each other, are split, a change in one affects the other *simultaneously* – no matter how far apart they are. This instantaneous, non-local connection goes beyond any conventional notion of information transfer. It all seems beyond comprehension, and scientists still cannot explain it other than saying that even though they are physically separated, an invisible, connecting 'something' keeps them linked. Many scientists refer to 'hidden variables' as the answer, although Einstein himself stated that empty space contains enough 'vacuum energy' to exert outward pressure on the universe, and that particles cannot be separated from the space that surrounds them. They are all one. The One-ness, or Allness, composed of somethingness and nothingness, is the spirit of God. Time and space are not separate. It is only our perceptions of time and space that make parts of the Allness seem separate.

We can be aware of this in the subtlest of ways when we meditate, and when we attempt to uncover our levels of awareness. For example, when I observe what is happening around me, I am aware. When I think about what I have observed, I am aware that I am aware. When I contemplate my awareness, I become aware of my being aware that I am aware. If I continue in this way, I soon reach a point beyond which I cannot be aware of being aware that I am aware of being aware that I am aware. It's a bit like sitting in front of a mirror, looking at your reflection in the mirror behind you, and seeing the same picture repeated again and again and again.

I believe the synchronous and co-existent nature of Allness also reveals itself to us through flashes of intuition and through coincidence. Unfortunately, we are often so preoccupied or distracted, that it becomes difficult to hear or respond to the voice of me-in-God and God-in-me. This truth has been known for ages. In the Ghita, Krishna says us that if you see yourself in all and all in you, then you know reality; in ancient Greece, Protagoras said,' Man is the measure of all things.'

There are things of which we can be aware and others of which we cannot, so we need to be mindful that even though events may, and will, overtake us, we can choose the way in which we respond. In doing so, we confirm the paradox that free will and fate can exist side by side. Free will is reflected in the courage I show when I change the things I can; Fate is reflected in the serenity I display in accepting the things I cannot change. The wisdom I have to know the difference I derive from God.

Life demands that we answer its call. Life expects us to reciprocate. In exchange for the gift of life, we must give life a gift, some act of creation that underlines our existence and our presence, now and in the future: a child, a book, a score of music, a work of art, an act of love, a life fulfilled. The moment you become aware of your responsibility to life, and accept that every moment is a new beginning, you will never want to throw away this precious gift. As the philosopher Friedrich Nietszche said, 'He who has a why to live for can bear almost any how.' If you can accept that death can occur at any time, even if you do not have a life-threatening disease, then you will appreciate that you have prepared for death so it never comes as a surprise. The need for this preparation is highlighted in the tale told by Sai Baba, of an Indian holy man, the master of the house, who was dying. His wife and children pestered him with their anxiety. 'What is to happen to us, when you leave us?' they wailed.

In equal despair, the dying man turned to them. 'What is to happen to me, when I leave you?' he asked, and then died.

Baba goes on to say, 'Do not move helplessly on, to that doom of despair. Do not die in spirit, though the body man falls away. Know that the real "You" is deathless; make death a sublime act of liberation.' [9]

It is the central theme of this book that survivors are people who understand what is happening to them, face up to the challenge of a life-threatening disease, and discover the wisdom of God woven into the fabric of their body and soul.

A life-threatening disease gives us all a unique opportunity to prepare for death, to discover that in preparing to die, we get more out of life and, as with drawing up a living will, knowing that once you have taken care of your dying, you are free to live, in the knowledge that, as the Sioux Indians say, 'Every day is a good day to die.'

Life is intrinsically precious. We have value in being, not just in doing. Our way through life and our survival depends on our conviction that we are worthy of this life, and that nothing can be regarded as valuable unless it is assessed in relation to something higher in value. I was – am still – reminded of the sage words of Sai Baba, the Indian holy man, who wrote, 'Man knows how many seeds there are in an apple. Only God knows how many apples there are in a seed.'

Life lived as an event is a drama; reduced to a process, it becomes vegetation. Our awareness of life as a drama comes about as a result of knowing that we have a part to play, realising that the self is unprecedented, and refusing to regard existence as a waste. Being human involves being sensitive to the sacred.[10]

The white light of eternity awaits us all, and the struggle to make it through continues. If you have a passionate love for life, and the courage to rise to its challenges, remember the words of the Swahili Warrior Song:

Life has meaning only in the struggle;
Triumph or defeat is in the hands of the Gods.
So, let us celebrate the struggle.

We have to die to discover life is indestructible, and death the link we need to close the circle. God prevents us from predicting the future so we are forced to live in today. In truth, you cannot fear death nor bemoan the brevity of life when you recognise that your essence is timeless, and death is only of the body that encased a blessed part of the mind of God.

Part Five

notes and

resources

notes

☙

CHAPTER TWO   Understanding your diagnosis

1   Jean Aitken-Swan and E.C. Easson, 'Reactions of Cancer Patients on being told of their Diagnosis', *British Medical Journal*, March 21 1959, pp. 779–83.

2   National Health & Medical Research Council, *General Guidelines for Medical Practitioners On Providing Information to Patients*, Commonwealth of Australia, 1993.

3   Elisabeth Kübler-Ross, *Living with Death and Dying*, Souvenir Press, London, 1988.

4   'How we Feel', in *A Consumer Prescription for the Health System*, National Consumer Affairs Advisory Council, Australian Government Publishing Service, Canberra, December 1992.

5   Franz J. Inglefinger, 'Arrogance', *New England Journal of Medicine*, 303, 26 (1980), pp. 1507–11.

CHAPTER THREE   Breaking the news

1   Allan Kellehear, *Dying of Cancer: The Final Year of Life*, Harwood, Chur, 1990, pp. 95–8.

2   Tessa Wilkinson, *The Death of a Child*, Julie MacRae Books, London, 1991, pp. 19–21.

3   Dan Schaeffer and Christine Lyons, *How do we tell the children?*, Newmarket Press, New York, 1988, pp. 30–2; David Spiegel, *Living Beyond Limits*, Fawcett Columbine, New York, 1993, pp. 209–18; *American Cancer Society, Helping Children Understand*, American Cancer Society Inc., 1986; *Explaining Death to Children*, ed. Earl Grollman, Beacon Press, Boston, 1967, pp. 106–8.

4   *Explaining Death to Children*, op.cit.; Schaeffer and Lyons, op.cit.; Earl A. Grollman, *Straight Talk About Death For Teenagers*, Beacon Press, Boston, 1993, pp. 91–3; Ernest Becker, *The Denial of Death*, The Free Press, New York, 1973; D.W. Winnicott, *The Child, The Family, and the Outside World*, Penguin, Harmondsworth, 1964, pp. 85–110;

R. M. Youngson, *Grief: Rebuilding Your Life after Bereavement*, David
& Charles, Newton Abbot, 1989; American Cancer Society Inc., op.cit.
5 Schaeffer and Lyons, op.cit., pp. 82–7; Becker, op.cit.
6 Schaeffer and Lyons, op.cit.
7 Doris Buchanan Smith, *A Taste of Blackberries*, Penguin,
Harmondsworth, 1987, p. 70.
8 Alice Miller, *For Your Own Good*, Virago, London, 1990.
9 Schaeffer and Lyons, op.cit., pp. 94–9.

CHAPTER FOUR The right doctoring
1 M. Tattersal et al., 'Undergraduate Education about Cancer. A Survey
of Clinical Oncologists and Clinicians responsible for Cancer Teaching in
Australian Medical Schools', *Cancer Forum*, Australian Cancer Society,
18, 1 (March, 1994), pp. 24–7.
2 'How We Feel: A Consumer Prescription for the Health System',
National Consumers Affairs Advisory Council, Canberra, December
1992.
3 Kübler-Ross, op.cit.
4 Nira Kfir and Maurice Slevin, *Challenging Cancer: from chaos to control*,
Routledge, London, 1991.
5 Aitken-Swan and Easson, op.cit.; Kline & Sobin, 'The Psychological
Management of Cancer Cases', *Journal of the American Medical Association*,
146, 17 (1951), pp. 1547–1551; Donald Oken, 'What to Tell Cancer
Patients', *Journal of the American Medical Association*, 175, 13 (1961),
pp. 86–94; Stuart E. Lind et al., 'Telling the Diagnosis of Cancer', *Journal
of Clinical Oncology*, (USA), 7, (1989), pp. 583–9; John Hinton, 'Whom do
Dying Patients tell?', *British Medical Journal*, 281 (1980), pp. 1328–30;
Catherine Meredith et al., 'Information Needs of Cancer Patients in West
Scotland: Cross Sectional Survey of Patients' Views.', *British Medical
Journal*, 313, 7059 (1996), pp. 724–6; 'General Guidelines for Medical
Practitioners on Providing Information to Patients', National Health and
Medical Research Council, Commonwealth of Australia, Canberra, 1993.

CHAPTER FIVE How to be a survivor
1 D.H. Bovbjer, 'Psychoneuroimmunology. Implications for Oncology?',
Cancer (USA), 67, 3 (1991), Suppl. 1, pp. 823–32; J.S. McDaniel,
'Psychoimmunology: implications for future research', *Southern Medical
Journal* (USA), 85, 4 (1992), pp. 388–96, 402; R. Glaser and J. Kiecolt-
Glaser (eds), *Handbook of Human Stress and Immunity*, Academic Press,
San Diego, 1994; D. Spiegel et al., 'Effect of psychosocial treatment on

survival of patients with metastatic breast cancer', *Lancet*, 2, 8668 (1989), pp. 888–91.

2 John Hinton, *Dying*, Penguin, Harmondsworth, 1990.

3 Dennis A. Casciato and Barry B. Lowitz (eds) *Manual of Clinical Oncology*, 3rd edn, Little, Brown, Boston, 1995.

4 M. Maltoni et al., 'Predictions of Survival of Patients Terminally Ill with Cancer,' *Cancer* (USA), 75 (1995), pp. 2613–62.

5 Stanley Cohen and Laurie Taylor, *Psychological Survival*, Penguin, Harmondsworth, 1981.

6 Steven Callahan, *Adrift: 76 Days Lost at Sea*, Ballantine, New York, 1996.

7 Viktor E. Frankl, *The Doctor in the Soul*, Vintage, New York, 1986.

8 Hinton, Dying, op.cit.; Cohen & Taylor, op.cit.; Frankl, op.cit.; Bruno Bettelheim, *Surviving and Other Essays*, Thames and Hudson, London, 1979; Viktor Frankl, *Man's Search for Meaning*, Washington Square Press, New York, 1984; Hilde O. Bluhm, 'How did they Survive? Mechanisms of Defence in Nazi Concentration Camps,' *American Journal of Psychology*, 2 (1948), pp. 3–32.

9 H.S. Greer et al., 'Psychological Response to Breast Cancer: Effect on Outcome,' *Lancet*, 2 (1979), pp. 785–787.

10 L.R. Derogatis et al., 'Psychological Coping Mechanisms and Survival in Metastatic Breast Cancer,' *Journal of American Medical Association*, 242 (1979), pp. 1504–8; S. Levy et al., 'Breast Conservation v. Mastectomy', *Journal of Clinical Oncology* (USA), 7 (1989), pp. 367–75; J.K. Kiecolt-Glaser et al., 'Distress and DNA Repair in Human Lymphocytes,' *Journal of Behavioral Medicine* (USA), 8 (1985), pp. 311–20.

CHAPTER SIX Weighing up alternatives

1 Kübler-Ross, op.cit.

2 Hinton, *Dying*, op.cit.

3 Lynne McTaggert, 'Cures for Cancer', *WellBeing* (Australia), Collectors' Edition, 1995 Annual, p. 27.

4 M.J. Massie and J.C. Holland, 'Overview of Normal Reactions and Prevalence of Psychiatric Disorders,' in *Handbook of Psycho-oncology: Psychological Care of the Patient with Cancer*, ed. J.C. Holland and J.H. Rowland, Oxford University Press, New York, 1989, pp. 273–82; A.D. Weisman and J.W. Worden, 'The Existential Plight in Cancer: Significance of the First 100 Days', *International Journal of Psychiatry in Medicine* (USA), 7, 1 (1956), pp. 1–15; John Hinton, *Dying*, op.cit.; *The Merck Manual of Diagnosis & Therapy*, 16th edn, Merck, Rahway,

N.J., 1992, pp. 1625–6; M.J. Massie and E.J. Shakin, 'Management of Depression and Anxiety in Cancer Patients,' in *Psychiatric Aspects of Symptom Management in Cancer Patients*, ed. W. Breitbart and J. C. Holland, American Psychiatric Press, Washington, 1993, pp. 470–91.
5 Medical Tribune News Service, USA, 8 February 1996; William J. Blot et al., 'Nutrition intervention trials in Linxian, China: Supplementation with Specific Vitamin/mineral Combinations, Cancer Incidence, and Disease-specific Mortality in the General Population,' *Journal of the National Cancer Institute* (USA), 85 (1993), pp. 1483–92; O. P. Heinonen and D. Albanes, 'The Effect of Vitamin E and Beta Carotene on the Incidence of Lung Cancer and Other Cancers in Male Smokers. The Alpha-Tocopherol, Beta-Carotene Cancer Prevention Study Group,' *New England Journal of Medicine*, 330, 15 (1994), pp. 1029–35.
6 American Cancer Society, *Cancer Facts and Figures 1994*, Atlanta, 1994; John C. Bailar III and Heather L. Gornik, 'Cancer Undefeated', *The New England Journal of Medicine*, 336, 22 (1997), pp. 1569–74; D. M. Parkin et al., 'Estimates Of the Worldwide Frequency of Sixteen Major Cancer Cancers in 1980', *International Journal of Cancer* (USA), 41(1988), p. 107.
7 Robert N. Proctor, *Cancer Wars: How Politics Shapes What We Know and Don't Know About Cancer*, Basic Books, New York, 1995; Dept. of Human Services and Health, *Cancer Control in Australia. A review of current activities and future directions*, Australian Government Publishing Service, Canberra, 1995, pp. 1–10.
8 P. Jelfs, M. Coates, G.Giles et al., 'Cancer in Australia: 1989–90 (with Projections to 1995), *Australian Institute of Health and Welfare: Cancer Series*, No. 5, Australian Government Publishing Service, Canberra, 1996; *Age*, Melbourne, Australia, 7 January, 1994.
9 Annette & Richard Bloch, *Fighting Cancer*, Bloch Cancer Foundation, Kansas City, 1985; Department of Human Services and Health, op.cit., pp. 68–70 and 74–5.
10 Proctor, op.cit.
11 Department of Human Services and Health, op.cit.
12 P.A. Singer et al., 'Sex or Survival: Trade-Offs Between Quality and Quantity of Life', *British Journal of Oncology*, 9, 2 (1991), pp. 328–34.
13 L. Tomatis (ed.), 'Cancer: Causes, occurrence and control: World Health Organisation International Agency for Research on Cancer', *IARC Scientific*, Lyon, 1990; W.C. Willett and D. Trichopoulos, 'Summary of the evidence: Nutrition and Cancer' in 'Cancer Causes and Control. An International Journal of Studies of Cancer in Human Populations', *Official Journal of the International Association of Cancer Registries*, 7, 1

(1996), Rapid Science, London, pp. 3–4 and 178–9; Public Affairs and
Behavioral Intervention Committee, 'Cancer Control in Australia:
A Review of Current Activities and Future Directions', Australian
Government Publishing Service, Canberra, 1995: Anton Bonett, Paul
Dickman et al., 'Survival of Cancer Patients in South Australia, 1977–90,
South Australian Health Commission, Adelaide, 1992.

14 J. H. Knowles (ed.), *Doing Better and Feeling Worse: Health in the United
States*, Norton, New York, 1977.

15 J. Personett, 'Bacterial Infection as a Cause of Cancer: Environment
Health Perspective', Departments of Medicine & Health Research &
Policy, 103, 8 (1995), Stanford, pp. 263–8.

16 C. Ip et al., 'Mammary Cancer Prevention by Conjugated Dienopic
Derivative of Linoleic Acid', *Cancer Research* (USA), 51 (1991),
pp. 6118–24.

17 Medical Tribune News Service, 8 February, 1996; J. Blot, op.cit.;
Alpha-Tocopherol, Beta-Carotene Study, op.cit.

18 S. Wheeler and Peter Selby, *Confronting Cancer: Cause and Prevention*,
Penguin, London, 1993.

CHAPTER SEVEN   Treatment options

1   Willett and Trichopoulos, op.cit.

2   Kent Nelson Tigges and William Matthew Marcil, *Terminal and Life
Threatening Illness. An Occupational Behaviour Perspective*, Slack,
Thorofare, N.J., 1988.

3   R. Demicheli et al., 'Time Distribution of the Recurrence Risk for
Breast cancer Patients undergoing Mastectomy: Further Support about
the Concept of Tumor Dormancy', *Breast Cancer Research Treatment*,
(USA), 41, 2 (1996), pp. 177–85.

4   *Merck Manual of Diagnosis and Therapy*, op.cit.

5   Jack Thomas (ed.), *Australian Prescription Products Guide*, Australian
Pharmaceutical Publishing Co. Ltd., Melbourne, 1994; Dennis Albert
Cadsciato, and Barry Bennet Lowitz (ed.), *Manual of Clinical Oncology*,
Little, Brown, Boston, 1991; *Merck Manual of Diagnosis and Therapy*, op cit.

6   V. Anku, *What to know about the treatment of cancer*, Madrona
Publishers, Seattle, 1984.

7   *Merck Manual of Diagnosis and Therapy*, op.cit., pp. 1275–77.

8   Thomas, *Australian Prescription Products Guide*, op.cit.; *Manual of
Clinical Oncology*, op.cit.; *Merck Manual of Diagnosis and Therapy*, op.cit.

9   E.T. Creagan et al., 'Randomised Surgical Adjuvant Clinical Trial of
Recombinant Interferon alfa-2a in Selected Patients with Malignant

Melanoma', *Journal of Clinical Oncology* (USA), 13, 11 (1995), pp. 2776–83; D. Reintgen and J. Kirkwood, 'The adjuvant treatment of malignant melanoma,' Journal of Florida Medical Association, 84, 3 (1997), pp. 147–52.

10 Vincent T. De Vita Jnr et al., (ed.), *CANCER. Principles & Practice of Oncology*, 3rd ed., J.B. Lippincott , Philadelphia, 1991.

11 Steven A. Rosenberg, *The Transformed Cell. Unlocking the Mysteries of Cancer*, Chapmans, London, 1992, pp. 249–56.

12 'Stopping Cancer in it tracks,' Time, 25 April 1994.

13 J. Vieweg and E. Giboa, 'Gene Therapy Approaches in Urologic Oncology,' *Surgical Oncology Clinics of North America*, 4, 2 (1995), pp. 203–18; Creagan et al., op.cit.

14 P.W. Laird et al., 'Suppression of Intestinal Neoplasia by DNA Hypomethylation,' *Cell* (USA), 81, 2 (1995), pp. 197–205.

15 Robert Castleberry and Peter Emanuel, 'A Pilot Study of Isotretinoin in the Treatment of Juvenile Chronic Myelogenous Leukemia', *New England Journal of Medicine*, 331, 25 (1994), pp. 1680–4.

16 Vincent T. De Vita Jnr. et al., (ed.), *Cancer: Principles & Practice of Oncology*, 3rd edn., Lippincott, Philadelphia, 1991; Ralph W. Moss, 'Phototherapy', in *Cancer Therapy*, Equinox Press, New York, 1993, pp. 386–95; J.F. Evensen, 'The use of Porphyrins and Non-ionizing Radiation for Treatment of Cancer', *Acta Oncology* (USA), 34, 8 (1995), pp. 1103–10; M.A. Biel, 'Photodynamic Therapy of Head and Neck Cancers', *Seminars in Surgical Oncology* (USA), 11, 5 (1995), pp. 355–9.

17 H. Jablonowski et al., 'Long-term use of DOX-SL (Stealth Liposomal Doxorubicin HCl) in the Treatment of Moderate to Severe AIDS-related Kaposi's Sarcoma', Proceedings of the Annual Meeting of the American Society of Clinical Oncologists, 15, A842 (1996).

18 L.D. Mayer et al., 'Pharmacology of Liposomal Vincristine in Mice Bearing L1210 Ascitic and B16/BL6 Solid Tumors', *British Cancer Journal*, 71, 3 (1995), pp. 482–8.

19 Danilo Lasic, 'Liposomes,' in *Science & Medicine*, (Philadelphia), May/June, 1996.

20 'Gene Therapy for Cancer. A Special Report', in *Scientific American*, New York, June 1997.

CHAPTER EIGHT Side effects of treatment

1 *Merck Manual of Diagnosis and Therapy*, op.cit.

2 National Health & Medical Research Council, *The Management of Severe Pain*, Australian Government Publishing Service, Canberra, 1988, pp. 4 and 29.

3 Ronald Melzack, 'The Tragedy of Needless Pain', in *Scientific American* special issue on Medicine, New York, 1993.

4 Tigges and Marcil, op.cit.

5 C.S. Cleeland et al., 'Pain and Its Treatment in Outpatients with Metastatic Cancer', *New England Journal of Medicine*, 330, 9 (1994), pp. 592–6; Correspondence: 'Treating Cancer Pain' in *New England Journal of Medicine*, 331, 3 (1994), pp. 199–200; World Health Organisation, Cancer Pain Relief, 1996; Kathleen M. Foley, 'Controlling the Pain of Cancer' in *Scientific American*, special issue, New York, September 1996.

6 National Health & Medical Research Council, op.cit.

7 Larry Dossey, *Space, Time & Medicine*, Shambhala, Boston, 1982.

8 H.S. Kaplan, 'A Neglected Issue: The Sexual Side Effects of Current Treatments for Breast Cancer,' *Journal of Sex and Marital Therapy* (USA), 18, 1 (1992), pp. 3–19.

CHAPTER NINE What are your rights?

1 William Shakespeare, *Macbeth*, Act 1, Scene iii.

2 David Lanham, *Taming Death by Law*, Longman, Melbourne, 1993.

3 Sue Parker, 'More than a Silent Witness', in *Nursing Times* (UK), 19–25 March 1997; C. Game et al., 'Legal Principles in the Practice of Medical Surgical Nursing', in *Medical Surgical Nursing: A Core Text*, Churchill Livingstone, Melbourne, 1989, pp. 21–32.

4 J. Benson and N. Britten, 'How Much Truth and to Whom? Respecting the Autonomy of Cancer Patients when Talking with their Families: Ethical Theory and the Patient's View,' *British Medical Journal*, 313, 7059 (1996), pp. 729–31.

5 National Health and Medical Research Council, op.cit.; Robert Buckman, 'Talking to patients about cancer' editorial, *British Medical Journal*, 313, 7059 (1996), pp. 699–700.

6 'How We Feel', op.cit., pp. 41–2.

7 Lanham, op.cit. pp. 41–3.

8 J.F. Holland et al., 'Adjuvant Chemotherapy for Breast Cancer with 3 or 5 drugs, CMF v CMFVP', in *Proceedings of the American Association of Cancer Research and American Association of Surgical Oncologists*, 22 (1981), p. 386.

9 Lanham, op.cit., p. 4; T. Patrick Hill and David Shirley, *A Good Death*, Addison Wesley, Reading, 1992; Derek Humphrey, *Final Exit*, Penguin Books, Harmondsworth, 1991; Judith Ahronheim and Doron Weber, *Final Passages*, Simon & Schuster, New York, 1992.

10 Lanham, op.cit.

11 Joni Eareckson Tada, *When is it right to die?*, Zondervan, South
Barrington, 1992.

12 J.P. Orlowski et al., 'Pediatric Euthanasia', *American Journal of Diseases
of Children*, 146, 12 (1992), pp. 1440–6; G. Van der Wal and R. Dillman,
'Euthanasia in the Netherlands', *British Medical Journal*, 308, 6940 (1994),
pp. 1346 –9; F.G. Miller et al., in Sounding Board: 'Regulating Physician-
Assisted Death', *The New England Journal of Medicine*, 2, 331 (1994),
pp. 119–23.

13 Cicely Saunders, 'Into the Valley Of the Shadow of Death: On A
personal therapeutic journey,' *British Medical Journal*, 13, 7072 (1996),
pp. 1599–1600.

14 Lanham, op.cit.

15 Washington v. Glucksberg, 96–110, 1997 WL 348094, US Supreme
Court, 26 June, 1997, quoting New York State Task Force on 'Life and
the Law, When Death is Sought: Assisted Suicide and Euthanasia in the
Medical Context', (1994) at 120.

16 Washington Revised Code §70.122.070 (1) [n.2] 1979, in Washington
v. Glucksberg, op.cit.

17 Reported in 'Physician Assisted Suicide and Euthanasia in the
Netherlands', A Report of Chairman Charles T. Canady to the
Subcommittee on the Constitution of the House Committee on the
Judiciary, 104th Congress, 2nd Session, 10–11, Committee Print,
Washington, 1996.

18 Tada, op.cit.

19 Lanham, op.cit., pp. 11–14 and 44–6.

CHAPTER TEN Understanding feelings

1 Elisabeth Kübler-Ross, *On Death and Dying*, Tavistock, London, 1970.

2 Kellehear, *Dying of Cancer*, op.cit., pp. 19–22.

3 Kübler-Ross, op.cit.

4 Allan Kellehear and Jan Fook, Sociological Factors in Death Denial by
the Terminally Ill, Unpublished MS, 1991, pp. 1–20.

5 J. Hackett, 'The Coronary Care Unit: An Appraisal of Its Psycholgical
Hazards', *New England Journal of Medicine*, 279, 1365 (1968), reported by
Larry Dossey in Meaning and Medicine, op.cit.

6 Elisabeth Kübler-Ross, *Living with Death and Dying*, Souvenir Press,
London, 1981; Bernie S. Siegel, *Peace, Love and Healing*, Harper & Row,
New York, 1989.

A similar version of this story appears in both of these books. It seems
immaterial as to who first told it as it so aptly illustrates the very real and

positive aspect of using bargaining to set future goals as a life-enhancing process.

7 Becker, *The Denial of Death*, op.cit.
8 R. Buckman, *How to break bad news*, Macmillan, London, 1991.
9 Grollman, *Straight Talk About Death For Teenagers*, op.cit.

CHAPTER ELEVEN   Living with cancer
1 Kübler-Ross, *On Death and Dying*, op.cit.
2 This information is derived from article written by Joel Nathan which first appeared in *Private Health Choice*, (Australia), 4, 1994.
3 Bill Moyers, *Healing and the Mind*, Doubleday, New York, 1993; D. Spiegel et al., op.cit.

CHAPTER TWELVE   Restoring balance in your life
1 J. Licinio et al., 'The molecular mechanism for stress-induced alterations in susceptibility to disease,' *Lancet*, 346, 8967 (1995), pp. 104–6; Bovbjer, op.cit.; McDaniel, op.cit. ; J.K. Kiecolt-Glaser et al., 'Endocrine and Immune Function,' in *Handbook of Human Stress and Immunity*, ed. R. Glaser and J. Kiecolt-Glaser, San Diego Academic Press, San Diego, 1994.
2 Esther M. Sternberg, 'The Stress Response & the Regulation of Inflammatory Disease', *Annals of Internal Medicine* (USA), 117, 10 (1992), pp. 854–66; J. Licinio et al., 'The Molecular Mechanism for Stress-induced Alterations in Susceptibility to Disease,' *Lancet*, 346 (1995), pp. 104–6.
3 Bill Moyers, *Healing and the Mind*, Doubleday Publishing, USA, 1993; Arthur Janov, *The New Primal Scream*, Cardinal Books, London, 1992; Alice Miller, *Breaking Down the Wall of Silence*, Virago, London, 1991.
4 Ainslie Meares, *Dialogue on Meditation*, Hill of Content, Melbourne, 1979.
5 Merck, op.cit., pp. 1266–7 and 2294–5.
6 Ashley Montagu, *On Being Human*, Abelard-Schuman, London, 1957.
7 Zerrin Pelin, 'Sleep Deprivation Affects Immune Cells, Department of Neurology Sleep Disorders Unit of Istanbul University Cerrahpasa Medical School', Report by Reuters Limited, New York, 17 June 1997; Michael Irwin, John McClintick et al., 'Partial night sleep deprivation reduces natural killer and cellular immune responses in humans,' *Journal of Federation of America Societies of Experimental Biology*, 10, 5 (1966), pp. 643–53.
8 Samuel H. Dresner (ed.), *I asked for Wonder: A spiritual anthology of Abraham Heschel*, Crossroad, New York, 1990.

9 David Bohm, *Wholeness and the Implicate Order*, Ark Paperbacks, London, 1983, p.xv.
10 Spiegel, *Living beyond limits*, op.cit.

CHAPTER THIRTEEN Living in the face of death

1 Carl Jung, 'The Development of the Personality', in *Collected Works of Carl Jung*, 17, Routledge & Kegan Paul, London, 1953, pp. 299f.
2 William J. Schwartz, 'Internal Timekeeping' in *Science & Medicine*, Philadelphia, May/June 1996, pp. 44–53.
3 Robert H. Schuller, *Tough Times Never last, But Tough People Do*, Bantam, New York, 1984.
4 Cohen and Taylor, op.cit.
5 Bettelheim, *Surviving and Other Essays*, op.cit.
6 Kenneth Ring, *Heading Towards Omega: In Search of the Meaning of the Near Death Experience*, William Morrow, New York, 1985; Kenneth Ring, *Life at Death: A Scientific Investigation of the Near-Death Experience*, Coward, MCann and Geoghegan, New York, 1980; Raymond Moody, *Life after Life*, Bantam, New York, 1984; Carol Zaleski, *Other World Journeys*, Oxford University Press, New York, 1987.
7 Frankl, *The Doctor in The Soul*, op.cit.
8 Frankl, *Man's Search for Meaning*, op.cit.
9 Sai Baba, *Sathya Sai Speaks*, Volume 2, Sri Sathya Sai Education Foundation, New Delhi (1970).
10 Abraham J. Heschel, *God in search of Man*, The Noonday Press, New York, 1955.

resource guide

There are cancer councils and associations in over 85 countries around the world. Some offer more comprehensive services than others; however, since almost all are members of the International Union Against Cancer (UICC), they can contact each other. So there is no shortage of places from which you can gain additional information to enable you to make choices about ways to improve the quality of your life or to ensure you get the best medical treatment and follow-up services. You can find out about your particular type of cancer and about support groups, visiting services, counselling – or obtain booklets, leaflets and recommended reading lists of books dealing with all aspects of cancer. The best cancer councils can also tell you about the latest clinical trials – where they are being conducted and how to contact the relevant hospital or institute – and either can provide you with a living will, enduring power of attorney or value inventory, or tell you where these can be obtained.

CANCER ASSOCIATIONS

Some countries have a single telephone number you can call toll-free or for the cost of a local call no matter where you live. For example,

- AUSTRALIA: Cancer Helpline (throughout all of Australia) 13 11 20 (in Queensland call 1300 361 366).
- CANADA: Cancer Information Service (throughout all of Canada) 1-888-939-3333.
- USA: Cancer Information Service (throughout all of the USA) 1-800-4-CANCER.
  Cancer Care Inc. Counselling line (throughout USA) 1-800-813-HOPE.

Other countries do not offer these low-rate calls but do offer excellent facilities, for example:

- NEW ZEALAND: Cancer Society of New Zealand, Wellington Division (from anywhere in New Zealand): (4) 389 8421.
- UK: Bacup: (171) 696 90 03
- HONG KONG: Hong Kong Anti-Cancer Society: 814 0950
- INDIA: Indian Cancer Society: 22-202 9941
  Cancer Patients Aid Association: 22-269 8964

INTERNET

With the introduction of the Internet and e-mail, many more people can now access the kind of information previously only available through a library – and even what was available then is incomparable to what you can now find, and to what you will be able to find in the future. Many cancer councils have their own Web sites, and there are many institution – and research-based sites that can provide you with information.

I must stress the point that none of these should ever be seen as a substitute for seeing a cancer specialist: they are resource centres from which you can obtain additional information and help. Of course, having the latest information will help you (and your doctor) ensure you receive the most up-to-date treatment for your particular type and stage of cancer.

INTERNATIONAL SITES

Some of the best Internet sites I have found include:

- ONCOLINK: http://oncolink.upenn.edu/search/
- NATIONAL CANCER INSTITUTE (USA):
  http://cancernet.nci.nih.gov/patient.html
- MEDSCAPE: http://www.scp.com/medscape/html/medscape.html
- ONCOLOGY FORUM:
  http://www.oncology-forum.org/Patients/patframe.htm
- HEALTHFINDER: http://www.healthfinder.gov/search.htm

Some of the national cancer associations have excellent sites – for example:

- CANADA: http://www.bc.cancer.ca
- GERMANY: http://www.krebshilfe.de/krebshilfe
- ISRAEL: http://www.icl.co.il/c/cancer/

☞ Italy: http://www.legatumori.it
☞ UK: http://www.bacup.org.uk/
☞ USA: http://www.aacr.org
        http://www.asco.org

Australian sites

In Australia at this time there is no national cancer organisation Web site; however, the states are developing their own and most of these will direct you to the others. Try out

☞ New South Wales: http://www.nbcc.org.au
☞ Victoria: http://www.accv.org.au

As you will discover, the better Web sites provide 'hot links' to other sites so you can find the information most relevant to your search. Most Web sites list telephone, fax, and address details so you can contact them to find out even more.

Searching for information is one of the most positive steps you can take towards your goal of recovering from cancer. You open the door to new possibilities and many more choices when you work from the premise that understanding is a key to survival.

Values inventory

Contact your local cancer council or society for a copy of this invaluable form described in chapter 9. If they don't have a copy, they can obtain an original form, for a nominal fee, which they can then copy to their heart's content free of charge. They should contact:

Institute of Public Law
UNM School of Law
1117 Stanford NE
Albuquerque, NM 87131
USA

Tel: (505) 277-5006
Fax: (505) 277-7064

Information provided is accurate at time of printing.

index